Managing to Care

Case Management
and
Service System Reform

SOCIAL INSTITUTIONS AND SOCIAL CHANGE

An Aldine de Gruyter Series of Texts and Monographs

EDITED BY James D. Wright, *University of Central Florida*

V. L. Bengtson and W. A. Achenbaum, **The Changing Contract Across Generations**

Thomas G. Blomberg and Stanley Cohen (eds.), **Punishment and Social Control: Essays in Honor of Sheldon L. Messinger**

M. E. Colten and S. Gore (eds.), **Adolescent Stress: Causes and Consequences**

Rand D. Conger and Glen H. Elder, Jr., **Families in Troubled Times: Adapting to Change in Rural America**

Joel A. Devine and James D. Wright, **The Greatest of Evils: Urban Poverty and the American Underclass**

Ann E. P. Dill, **Managing to Care: Case Management and Service System Reform**

G. William Domhoff, **The Power Elite and the State: How Policy is Made in America**

G. William Domhoff, **State Autonomy or Class Dominance? Case Studies on Policy Making in America**

Paula S. England, **Comparable Worth: Theories and Evidence**

Paula S. England, **Theory on Gender/Feminism on Theory**

R. G. Evans, M. L. Barer, and T. R. Marmor, **Why Are Some People Healthy and Others Not? The Determinants of Health of Population**

George Farkas, **Human Capital or Cultural Capital? Ethnicity and Poverty Groups in an Urban School District**

Joseph Galaskiewicz and Wolfgang Bielefeld, **Nonprofit Organizations in an Age of Uncertainty: A Study in Organizational Change**

Davita Silfen Glasberg and Dan Skidmore, **Corporate Welfare Policy and the Welfare State: Bank Deregulation and the Savings and Loan Bailout**

Ronald F. Inglehart, Neil Nevitte, Miguel Basañez, **The North American Trajectory: Cultural, Economic, and Political Ties among the United States, Canada, and Mexico**

Gary Kleck, **Point Blank: Guns and Violence in America**

Gary Kleck, **Targeting Guns: Firearms and Their Control**

James R. Kluegel, David S. Mason, and Bernd Wegener (eds.), **Social Justice and Political Change: Public Opinion in Capitalist and Post-Communist States**

Theodore R. Marmor, **The Politics of Medicare** (Second Edition)

Thomas S. Moore, **The Disposable Work Force: Worker Displacement and Employment Instability in America**

Clark McPhail, **The Myth of a Madding Crowd**

James T. Richardson, Joel Best, and David G. Bromley (eds.), **The Satanism Scare**

Alice S. Rossi and Peter H. Rossi, **Of Human Bonding: Parent-Child Relations Across the Life Course**

Peter H. Rossi and Richard A. Berk, **Just Punishments: Federal Guidelines and Public Views Compared**

Joseph F. Sheley and James D. Wright: **In the Line of Fire: Youth, Guns, and Violence in Urban America**

David G. Smith, **Paying for Medicare: The Politics of Reform**

Linda J. Waite et al. (eds.), **The Ties That Bind: Perspectives on Marriage and Cohabitation**

Les G. Whitbeck and Dan R. Hoyt, **Nowhere to Grow: Homeless and Runaway Adolescents and Their Families**

James D. Wright, **Address Unknown: The Homeless in America**

James D. Wright and Peter H. Rossi, **Armed and Considered Dangerous: A Survey of Felons and Their Firearms** (Expanded Edition)

James D. Wright, Peter H. Rossi, and Kathleen Daly, **Under the Gun: Weapons, Crime, and Violence in America**

Mary Zey, **Banking on Fraud: Drexel, Junk Bonds, and Buyouts**

Managing to Care

Case Management
and
Service System Reform

Ann E. P. Dill

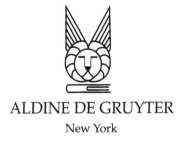

ALDINE DE GRUYTER

New York

ABOUT THE AUTHOR

Ann Dill, Associate Professor of Sociology and Gender Studies at Brown University, is a medical sociologist and social gerontologist. Her research examines issues affecting the long-term provision of health care and social services, both in the United States and in countries formerly part of Yugoslavia.

ALDINE DE GRUYTER
A division of Walter de Gruyter, Inc.
200 Saw Mill River Road
Hawthorne, New York 10532

This publication is printed on acid free paper ⊗

Library of Congress Cataloging-in-Publication Data

Dill, Ann E. P. 1948–
   Managing to care : case management and service system reform / Ann Dill.
      p. cm. — (Social institutions and social change)
   Includes bibliographical references and index.
   ISBN 0-202-30611-9 (cloth : alk. paper) — ISBN 0-202-30612-7 (pbk. : alk. paper)
   1. Social case work—Management.   2. Medical social work.
I. Title. II. Series.
   HV43 .D57 2001
   361.3'068—dc21   2001022601

Manufactured in the United States of America

10 9 8 7 6 5 4 3 2 1

CONTENTS

PREFACE AND ACKNOWLEDGMENTS

This book brings together thoughts developed over fifteen years of observing and participating in case management programs. It provides a multilayered perspective of case management, showing the linkages among its social and historical contexts and the ways it is practiced today in diverse service settings. My understanding of these complex relationships first emerged from several sets of comparatively simple observations.

My first set of insights came when I started my doctoral dissertation on the case management program for the "frail elderly" that I describe in Chapter 2. The literature on case management at that time, in the early 1980s, was full of the enthusiasm that suffuses new programs. Buoyed by the promises of what might be accomplished through better coordination of services, I was almost immediately deflated by the realities of the lives of clients case managers encountered in their work: lives with complicated, seemingly insoluble problems that coordination alone could barely salve. Lives, as well, of people determined to preserve their autonomy from the "experts." My respect for the case managers and their clients grew alongside my skepticism about relying too heavily on case management as an approach to service coordination.

A second set of observations came from more personal experiences some years later. As both my parents experienced major health crises, and especially as my mother endured her final illness, I realized the frustrations of all who try to preserve a sense of living normally and with integrity in the face of diminishing physical possibilities. A particular frustration was that my understanding of service fell short in application (even when joined with the knowledge of my physician brother). When dealing with multiple providers over multiple episodes of care, it became a full-time effort to work through systemic obstacles in order to weave a fabric of care that could sustain us all. While I emerged more than ever convinced about the essential need for care coordination, I also gained a clearer understanding of how our present ways of providing care can work against our highest objectives in doing so. This became a major theme for the book as I explored the paradoxes and contradictions embedded in case management practice.

More direct impetus for this book came from years of attending professional conferences in public health, gerontology, and social welfare, where I would hear firsthand the latest presentations of case management programs. As the philosophy of social policy governing our human services took a profound turn towards the right, the rhetoric of those presentations reflected a different discourse, one more concerned with costs and efficiency than before, while giving less voice to issues of access and advocacy. Curiously, the shape and structure of the programs remained largely intact. So, too, did explanations about the equivocal results that were achieved by those programs, which were explained almost entirely in technical terms such as those related to "sample selection," "target populations," and "comparison groups." While others also charted these trends, and a few began to trace their genesis, I found that most accounts of case management took for granted its origins, context, and status as a service technology.

The shape of this book began to appear as I struggled with the dilemmas presented by these different observations and experiences. Noting the convergence in issues affecting case management programs in different sectors, my friend and colleague David Rochefort, of Northeastern University, had suggested that I write a book comparing the history of case management in long-term care, mental health, and social welfare. Taking this as my basic framework, I tried then to unite my understandings of the history of human services, the organizational and professional practice of service delivery, and the experience of seeking care. Each chapter represents this union.

As with any project that encompasses years of study, many people contributed to and supported the work for this book. My first debt is to the case managers and clients who let me travel with them, sharing their lives and thoughts with unselfish openness. The diverse agencies, programs, and projects I represent here were equally generous in opening their doors, confident only that I would maintain their confidentiality and do my best to say something of meaning.

In bringing this book to light, I have been fortunate to receive intellectual guidance and patient prodding from valued colleagues, mentors, and friends. Jack Elinson and John Colombotos of Columbia University sponsored my first research on the subject. My work on mental health case management began during a postdoctoral fellowship at the Rutgers-Princeton Program in Mental Health Reseach, headed by David Mechanic. These three individuals have remained sources of support and inspiration. Phil Brown, Al Wessen, Gary Albrecht, and Jay Gubrium have provided close and thoughtful reviews of diverse portions of this work, in addition to consistent encouragement. I had the good fortune towards the end of this project to meet Yeheskel (Zeke) Hasenfeld, whose many writings on human services in general and case management in particular have enlivened and enlightened my thinking since the beginning of my work in this area. Carol Weiss, Bonnie Schorske, and Gayle Riesser of the New Jersey Division of Mental Health Services provided useful and timely commentary on Chapter 3. Thanks are due as well to countless classes of students who have reviewed the different bits and pieces of chapters I folded into lectures. David Rochefort must be singled out not merely for giving me the idea in the first place, but for never failing in thinking that it remained a good idea and that I was the person to see it through. Editorial and substantive guidance from Betty Levin, Martha Lang, and the members of my Women Writers group helped maintain my focus on the broader pictures, and especially those less often seen. Participants in the Course in Social Gerontology in International and Cross-Cultural Gerontology, held for years in Dubrovnik, Croatia, gave me the ideal feedback: that of people who, not sharing this society or culture, can question all our assumptions. Nada Smolić-Krkovíc, in particular, kept me centered on the heart, as well as the intellectual importance, of this work.

Support for the analysis and writing of this book came in part from the Henry Merritt Wriston Fellowship from Brown University. Funding for my initial research on case management programs, described in Chapter 2, came from a National Research Service Award from the National Institute of Mental Health (NIMH). The funding of my postdoctoral work on mental health case management (which informs Chapter 3) also came from the NIMH. The material on mental health clients presented in Chapter 3 derives from the Springfield Study of Populations with Disabilities (Susan M. Allen, P.I.), funded in part by the Robert Wood Johnson Foundation. Chapter 4 assesses material from interviews of social welfare recipients and officials in the Massachusetts Dept. of Public Welfare. David Rochefort and I conducted this research, which was named a "Better Government Competition Winner" in 1994 by the Pioneer Institute for Public Policy Research.

The physical work of production fell to many good hands. At the end, Berit Kosterlitz pulled the manuscript into order while Geoffrey Surrette made the figures come to life. Jan Goldsworthy and Christina Palaia eased the production process in every way imaginable. Jane Furth brought her keen eye to the typesetting, and Margaret Souza jumped in to help me figure out how to write a preface for a work emerging from a subject I have been interested in for almost one-third of my life. I have been grateful throughout to have excellent research assistants, including Kristen Peterson, Rick Harkins, and Kimberly Greene. Thanks, as well, to Peter DiPippo and Stephen Dill for easing the other strains and helping in at least a thousand ways.

Transcending categories of assistance, Richard Koffler provided exactly the right editorial guidance. As endless in his patience as acute in his reading, he stayed with me on a long course and helped make sure the book said what I wanted to say. The concluding chapter exists solely because of his suggestion, and I doubt the book would ever have been finished save for his help.

Beyond the usual disclaimer that all the flaws in this book are mine alone, I want to point out one that I identified late in the game and decided to keep for its heuristic value. As I presented some of the case material to a graduate seminar this past spring, I became aware that I had referred in a differential manner to the clients mentioned in Chapters 2, 3, and 4. In Chapter 2, representing elderly persons who received case management of home- and community-based services, I used fictitious surnames, e.g. "Mr. Valducci." When describing the clients of mental health case management in Chapter 3, I invented first names for the individuals who had been interviewed. In Chapter 4, I wrote about women who were receiving welfare payments, ascribing individual quotes to them but assigning them no names at all. What's in a name? In this case, my actions were in part due to the different contexts in which each piece of research had emerged and legacies of previous works I had published. Putting the three together, however, I ran into the discrepancy with some shock. I decided to keep things as they first emerged because I think my own biases here mirror those of society as well as human service systems in which I was doing research. Regarded with respect, if burdened with expectations of dependency, older people become distanced from the rest of us. Adults with chronic mental illness assume a different form of "other-hood," one where superficial familiarity collides with social stigma. Such stigma is even more pronounced for those on welfare, lumped without individual identity into a category of public and political opprobrium. For us to change these factors, we must first name them.

This book is highly critical of the ways case management has come to absorb and reflect the organizational flaws of the very service systems it was intended to reform. As the book's cover suggests, too often the management of the case comes to dominate the care. Nonetheless, I am not one to call for a rejection of professional systems in favor of a resurrected informal community. Such a stance tends to gloss cuts both in social programs and in our ability to know their results; it obscures, as well, the uncounted costs to families and particularly to women. While much can and should be done to strengthen our ties to one another, there will always be people whose problems require more expert help. I argue here that case management can provide such help, and provide it well, but only if grounded in the human dimension of a caring relationship. For giving me the fullest sense of what that can mean, I thank my parents and my son.

1

Introduction
What Is "the Case," and Why is It Managed?

Forged in response to social problems of human suffering, poverty, and distress, America's systems of health care and social welfare have themselves become social problems. Reforming those systems has led the domestic policy agenda and dominated front-page headlines throughout the past decade. National opinion polls in the 1990s found more Americans naming health care as the most important problem facing the country, save crime and violence, while the issue of welfare topped taxes, the environment, the trade deficit, and the international situation as an area of primary concern (Gallup, 1994). At its core, the public's sense of the problem is that these systems are out of control and we are paying for it, individually and collectively, with our money, our well-being, and even our lives.

The charges against human services are profound: that they are ineffective or inefficient, fragmented, uncoordinated, wasteful, and not affordable. The problems of service systems are also closely tied to much broader social concerns and controversies. Some of these address the actions of "players" and "payers": the role of the government versus the market; the administrative costs of insurance; the threatened autonomy of professional providers; the motives behind managed care. Yet others center on care recipients: Which groups are deserving and more (or more truly) needy than others? Which should be ineligible for a piece of the public pie?

The recent rounds of public debate on these issues rekindle much longer standing areas of discontent with the design and operation of human services. Over the three decades since present systems emerged from Great Society initiatives, policymakers, public administrators, and the public at large have actively pursued an array of programs attempting to bring those systems in line with desired goals. While the goals themselves have varied, from access and continuity in the 1960s and 1970s to coordination and cost constraint in the 1980s and 1990s, the constant expectation has been that the right reconfiguration of service systems can produce the right outcomes.

Case management has appeared throughout those decades as part of efforts to bring service systems into order and under control. Initially and still basically a tool for integrating services on the level of the individual client, case management has become a means of coordinating and rationalizing service delivery, rationing service resources, and constraining the costs of care. Short of the caring disciplines themselves, it is hard to think of a practice more widely distributed or accepted: In programs as diverse as public assistance, Medicaid, long-term care, mental health services, child welfare, care for people with AIDS, orthopedic rehabilitation, and services for the homeless, case management has become a fixture on the service landscape. It has found its way into health care and welfare reform proposals from proponents across the political spectrum and almost certainly will be central to any measures eventually adopted in the political arena. It would be easy to explain such remarkable and persistent popularity if case management were a clearly defined practice with a winning track record. This would require definite and agreed-upon standards about what it is, who should do it, and how it should be structured within particular organizations, as well as demonstrated success at achieving stated outcomes. Yet none of that is the case.

There is little consensus about the essential ingredients constituting case management, within, let alone across, service sectors. In long-term care, for example, there are presently no uniform state or federal standards for its practice, and three separate professional organizations have each developed standards which fall short of including specific performance guidelines with measurable outcome criteria (Geron & Chassler, 1994). In addition, case management has taken a variety of forms in different settings within and across sectors. In fact, the organizational structures, procedures, and personnel used under this rubric have been so diverse that one commentary in the mental health field likened case management to "a Rorschach test" onto which "an individual, agency, or a community will project ... its own particular solution to the problems it faces..." (Schwartz, Goldman, & Churgin, 1982, p. 1006). Because of this, it is difficult even to offer a comprehensive definition of the practice.

Moreover, the overall results of case management programs are consistent only in being strikingly ambiguous. In sector after sector, evaluation research outcomes vary from study to study and show at best modest gains from case management programs, often with offsetting deficits. Though assessing such outcomes is notoriously subject to bias from project and research design flaws, equivocal results emerge even from sophisticated, randomized control evaluations. Similarly, little conclusive evidence has accumulated about which forms or models of case management produce the best outcomes. Even the most systematic, experimental efforts to compare different types of programs yield few outcome differences, and those are as likely to disappoint as to validate the advocates of different approaches.

Why, then, has case management achieved such sustained and ubiquitous expansion as a feature of service systems? What accounts for the differences that have developed across and within service sectors? In what ways do case management programs accomplish their goals, and what helps them succeed? What happens when they fail? I contend that answers to these questions can be found by examining case management in social and historical context; that is, by understanding the social forces leading to the development of case management, the historical dynamics shaping it in particular sectors, and the social and organizational contexts in which case managers practice.

Case management has been the object of attention in the most significant trends in American health care and social welfare in the past quarter-century. It has also been one of the driving forces propelling those trends. These include the evolution and de-evolution of public bureaucracies; the challenging of once dominant professions; the shift from centralized institutional structures to community-based care; and the rise of corporate control, privatization, new technologies and professions, and managed care. To understand how case management has developed over time and in different sectors, we need to see it through a pinhole view of these forces transforming our human service systems and shaping particular programs. In turn, analyzing case management in this manner opens to scrutiny often taken-for-granted aspects of its practice and can help identify new possibilities for its application.

My purpose in this book is to explore the social history of case management strategies in order to examine critical service system issues and assess how case management practice reflects the social forces affecting systems, programs, and providers. I am particularly concerned with the symbolic as well as the structural basis of case management; that is, how the concepts, ideologies, and norms that define case management programs and practice are related to those shaping organizations, social systems, and society at large.

I have chosen to focus on three sectors which have relatively long histories of case management and which include among them particular case management approaches representing the range of practice found in other areas: long-term care, mental health, and welfare. Chapters 2 through 4 present historical and case study accounts of case management in each of these sectors. A major purpose in each chapter is to reveal the connections among the forces promoting case management programs, the historical environments in which they have developed, and the daily experience of case managers and their clients. To focus in on this last level, I draw from first-hand research on case management programs in each sector. This enables a comparative analysis of the dominant case management form or approach found in each: the "brokerage" model in long-term care, the "therapist" approach in mental health services, and the "gatekeeper" form of service management in welfare programs.

Looking across these sectors then prompts an examination, in Chapter 5, of recurrent issues in case management practice, program design, and standards. This review of other arenas—including care for people with AIDS, corporate programs, third-party payers, and private practice case management—leads to a critical discussion of the reasons for case management's continued popularity. Analyzing case management comparatively also opens to scrutiny what are often taken-for-granted aspects of its structure, and in particular the way it has been linked to the structures of gender, class, and race embedded in service systems. The chapter assesses the reasons for these connections and their significance for social policy and program design. Finally, the chapter explores the parallels and links between case management and managed care, illustrating as well the transformation in case management objectives from social casework to service management.

Chapter 6 concludes the book by assessing the strengths and limitations of the case management approach to service coordination, as well as ways in which it can be combined with broader-scale attempts at policy reform.

Before turning to the specific forms case management has taken in diverse sectors, we need to understand at a general level what it is and where it has come from. While it is difficult to offer a uniform definition of case management practice, it is possible to discern certain features crosscutting its diverse populations, goals, and structures. Similarly, the logic, objectives, and norms guiding case management in different settings have a common legacy in the origins of service systems. The next sections thus provide an overview of the distinguishing features and historical development of case management.

WHAT IS CASE MANAGEMENT?

An intervention using a human service professional to arrange and monitor an optimum package of services . . . (Applebaum & Austin, 1990, p. 5)

A set of logical steps and a process of interaction within a service network which assure that a client receives needed services in a supportive, effective, efficient, and cost effective manner. (Weil & Karls, 1985, p. 2)

A problem-solving function designed to ensure continuity of services and to overcome systems rigidity, fragmented services, misutilization of certain facilities and inaccessibility. (JCAH, 1976)

As these definitions imply, case management is less a concrete program than a service, a technology, a system, and a process (Bower, 1992). As a service provided to individual clients, case management includes many objectives: increasing their access to formal services, informing and assisting their decision making about service options, ensuring service continuity and integration, overseeing service effectiveness and productivity, and providing a human link to often impersonal systems.

Case management also encompasses the technology necessary to work toward those objectives. This includes the information, record-keeping, administrative, and evaluative systems needed to time, sequence, and coordinate complicated service programs for clients both individually and as a caseload. Not the least important component of case management technology is the role of case manager, the practitioner who (whether individually or as part of a team) bears the responsibility, authority, and accountability for managing the care of clients.

As a system, case management's functions encompass case identification, needs assessment, care plan development, service implementation and coordination, monitoring of clients and services over time, periodic reassessment of the client's condition, and adjustment or discontinuation of the service plan as appropriate. Regardless of the structure or components of specific case management programs, it is these functions that together comprise the essential elements of case management practice.

As recognized recently by the National Advisory Committee on Long-term Care Case Management, any one of these functions performed separately may be necessary to the success of a case management program, but does not in and of itself constitute that practice. The committee also acknowledged, as have previous analysts, that case management can also incorporate other functions to a greater or lesser degree, depending on the objectives to be served and the context of the program; these include outreach to identify clients, crisis intervention, counseling, advocacy on behalf of the client, and service development, or "class advocacy" (Geron & Chassler, 1994; see also Raiff & Shore, 1993).

Case management builds on established casework practice such as that found in nursing, social work, and some branches of medicine, elaborating a multifaceted and longitudinal process. The case manager simultaneously adopts an holistic view of client needs, organizes and coordinates care provided by multiple sources, and balances the task requirements of a caseload. Over time, the focus is on service episodes and changes in client needs. The locus of service delivery can cut across multiple settings, involving variable intensities, levels, and specialties of care (Bower, 1992).

While the operational goal of case management is to coordinate services at the level of individual clients, case management programs are also connected with multiple objectives related to the overall organization of ser-

Overall Objectives	**Goals for Clients**	**Goals for Service Systems**
	Timely, appropriate, integrated services of high quality, delivered in the least restrictive setting.	Promote service effectiveness, efficiency, quality, coordination, and cost containment.
Core Case Management Functions		
Case Finding and Needs Assessment	Enroll appropiate clients and establish service needs and preferences.	Provide appropriate and effective targeting of services.
Care Plan Development	Develop attainable service goals for and with clients.	Promote cost-effective care options. Restrict more costly and institutional care. Identify care gaps in service systems.
Service Implementation/Coordination	Ensure service access, delivery, continuity, and integration. Be the "human link" to the service system.	Enhance service system coordination, efficiency, and effectiveness. Advocate for service development to fill care gaps.
Monitoring and Adjusting Care Plan	Ongoing assesments of service need, delivery, and quality.	Provide quality assurance service outcomes. Promote better service targeting.

Figure 1. What Case Management Tries to Do: Goals for Clients and Service Systems

vice systems. Figure 1 illustrates how each of the core case management functions serves objectives for both clients and service systems.

Sometimes client- and system-level objectives represent different sides of the same goal. For example, many case management programs arose from attempts to construct a community-based care package in order to prevent or delay placement in institutional settings such as mental hospitals and nursing homes. On the systems' level, such efforts derived from interests in cost containment as well as concerns about the humaneness and quality of institutional care. For clients, preventing institutional care has the goals of promoting care in the least restrictive environment, enhancing quality of life, and encouraging self-care and independence (Bower, 1992).

On the other hand, the goals that case management programs seek for clients may conflict, or coexist in a dynamic tension, with those related to the functioning of service systems. For example, a common finding of case management programs in long-term care is that linking more clients with community-based services raises overall service expenditures even while offsetting institutionalization (Weissert, Cready, & Pawelak, 1988). Advocacy for particular cases may be in opposition to the organizational objective of ensuring broader interagency cooperation (Raiff & Shore, 1993).

The dual focus and complex, dynamic nature of case management reflect the complicated and changeable nature of the problems it attempts to address:

> Case management is a synergism evolving from the concern for humane care of the troubled, disabled, or sick individual combined with concern for the scientific management and conservation of community resources. It seems fair to speculate that case management would not exist if human problems were singular or simple, if they could be resolved with a single intervention, and if the needed interventions were readily available and inexpensive. (Weil & Karls, 1985, p. 10)

This said, it must also be acknowledged that case management has not come into existence simply because of the complexity of human problems and service systems. Case management has evolved in a particular social, historical context, the elements of which have fundamentally shaped its organization, operations, technology, and goals.

THE ORIGINS AND EVOLUTION OF CASE MANAGEMENT

Case management as a distinctive service component began as part of broader policy efforts to coordinate service systems. These efforts them-

selves evolved out of the concept of "service system" first developed in the
Progressive Era, then expanded through Great Society initiatives. Techniques of case management also have multiple origins, linked to early 20th
century welfare, social work, and nursing practice. To trace the history of
case management thus requires us to begin by examining the roots of our
service systems and their professions.

The System in "Service System"

Human service systems consist of organizations, institutions, providers,
payers, clients, and, perhaps most critically, ideas and principles about
how all these things should fit together and work as part of a system. In all
these areas, many parts of our current systems trace their origins to the period from the Civil War to the First World War. It is in this time that we find
the forebears to modern hospitals, pension systems, social service agencies, and public bureaucracies. This era also sees the beginning of the professional projects that would produce the current shape of medicine,
nursing, and social work. The organizational cultures of present service
systems—that is, the concepts, paradigms, and values that gird and guide
them—are the outgrowth of ideas, interests, and social movements of
those decades.

Two trends of this era have particular significance for the ancestry of
case management: the entrenchment of bureaucracy and the rise of dominant professions. Bureaucratic organization spread within and parallel to
the growth of capital industry in the late 19th century. Public, private, and
voluntary systems of health care and social welfare formed largely in response to the social dislocation and economic instability created by industrial expansion and the resulting phenomena of immigration and internal
migration (Quadagno, 1988; Haber & Gratton, 1994). Industry also provided the model of mechanical efficiency and productivity that became the
standard for bureaucratic systems, as evident in Weber's classic description:

> The decisive reason for the advance of bureaucratic organization has always
> been its purely technical superiority over any other form of organization. The
> fully developed bureaucratic mechanism compares with other organizations
> exactly as does the machine with the non-mechanical modes of produc-
> tion. . . . Precision, speed, unambiguity, knowledge of the files, continuity,
> discretion, unity, strict subordination, reduction of friction and of material
> and personal costs—these are raised to the optimum point in the strictly bu-
> reaucratic administration. (Weber, 1978, p. 973)

The human service professions developed in tandem with service bureaucracies in the early years of the 20th century. The movements of the

Progressive Era asserted not only the imperative of social reform but also "a technical and scientific elitism" (Lubove, 1975, p. 84) stressing the importance of professional expertise in defining and resolving social problems. In medicine, nursing, and social work there were collective efforts to garner the bodies of knowledge and corporate structures that are essential to the development of professional autonomy. In the process, professionals developed the technical and political coherence to define the operations, structures, and goals of service systems (see Bower, 1992; Greene, 1992; Larson, 1977; Lubove, 1975; Popple & Reid, 1999; Reverby, 1987; Starr, 1982).

From their beginnings, human service systems linked the structures, technologies, and models of bureaucracies with those of the helping professions in a symbolic as well as material manner. The logic and systems of classification that resulted would form a critical part of the rationale for case management. Basic elements of this included a focus on goals related to organizational productivity, a goal-driven or instrumental orientation, and categorical definitions of need applied at the level of the individual service recipient. Goals of efficiency, integration, coordination, and cost control are inherent in the mechanical paradigm of the service bureaucracy; they also provide the rhetoric identifying its flaws as those of inefficiency, fragmentation, and waste. Both bureaucratic and professional service activities depend on an instrumental goal orientation: They are designed to do something for or to an individual case. They further depend on controlling the categorical identification of need in that case; that is, having the ability to determine the fit between the case and the criteria for receiving the service product (whether a good, a form of care, or an indirect service such as a referral). Professional ideologies define need in terms of the theories and working knowledge that profession has developed as well as the services it can offer; service bureaucracies define need in terms of the regulations, policies, and procedures that specify their missions.

Since the 19th century days when a "charity agent . . . sat at a desk dividing the poor into categories of 'worthy' and 'unworthy'" (Lubove, 1975, p. 82), the categories of inclusion and exclusion used by service bureaucracies and professionals to classify those in need have changed (perhaps more than our social policy). It remains true, however, that the individual case is defined in terms of an individual person. In medicine and nursing, that definition has been part of the broader biomedical model identifying the individual as the unit of analysis (i.e., the patient) in the diagnosis and treatment of disease (Mishler et al., 1981). Although historically and ideologically involving more consideration of the social environment, social work has also focused on individual casework, especially since post–World War I shifts in theory and practice toward psychological and psychiatric paradigms (Lubove, 1975).

While professional systems convert distinct individual situations into differential diagnoses and treatment plans, service bureaucracies compress them into the basis for routinized official decisions as part of the rationalization and standardization needed to promote efficiency. Under both systems, cases that fail to fit within existing categories (whether of knowledge or of entitlement) are a problem. Since problems have already been defined as existing at the level of the individual, one likely response to individuals who are exceptions to the categories is to try to find a way to make an exception in practice, rather than to question the broader rationale of the categories themselves.

In the earliest antecedents to case management it is already possible to see a paradigm that frames the problems of service systems as those of fragmentation, lack of coordination, and waste, and that then attempts to remedy those problems through client-focused programs. In 1863, the state of Massachusetts charged the country's first board of charities with the coordination of public services for the poor and sick. The objective had a dual focus: "to assist the poor but also to guard the public coffers" (Weil & Karls, 1985, p. 4). Early settlement houses provided service coordination and advocacy for low-income and immigrant groups, using index card files to assemble information on families' social, educational, vocational, and environmental status and needs. The Charity Organization Societies (United Way forerunners that dominated human services from the end of the 1800s until the 1920s) maintained registries cross-checking the care families received from different organizations in order "to prevent cheating and duplication of assistance to the needy poor" (Carter, 1978, p. 2, cited in Weil & Karls, 1985, p. 5). In addition to these developments in the social services, public health programs at the turn of the century concerned themselves with community service coordination, provided at the client level by visiting nurses (Grau, 1984).

These early programs illustrate several operational elements and tensions that would later be built into case management. They served multiple objectives: documentation of need, program effectiveness, service advocacy, coordination of care, and resource accountability. Each attempted to find a balancing point in response to the "effectiveness-efficiency equation" (Weil & Karls, 1985, p. 4), recognizing that service agencies and systems had to operate efficiently in order to provide effective care to the greatest number of clients.

Like case management projects to come, the services these diverse programs offered were linked in a broad way to an objective of using community-based care as a more humane and less costly alternative to institutions of the almshouse and public hospitals (Haber & Gratton, 1994). The programs also had close ties within specific communities, and all faced multiple constituencies with interests in their work: clients and their families; neighborhood and ethnic associations; labor and industry organizations; politicians and public administrators; and service agencies and providers. While some oriented more toward the needs of their service counterparts and others emphasized advocacy and organizing on behalf of clients, all recognized the importance of interagency cooperation and coordination within community networks.

Emphasizing the need for systematic, client-focused coordination efforts, Mary Richmond, a leading figure in the Charity Organization Society movement and founder of social casework practice standards, developed what many consider the first formal precedent of case management. Richmond's model of the "forces with which the charity worker may cooperate" was client-centered and holistic, encompassing the client's informal resources (personal and familial), "neighborhood forces" (including neighbors, employers, the church, trade unions, social clubs, libraries, and banks), and formal institutions and services (civic bodies, private charitable resources, and "public relief") (Richmond, 1901, cited in Weil & Karls, 1985, pp. 6–7). The precepts and standards prompted by Richmond and other social service pioneers in turn fostered the basic building blocks of case management practice. These included instruments for comprehensively assessing client needs as well as the implementation of interagency and multidisciplinary case conferences.

Client-centered case coordination continued to be a service system theme into the middle of the 20th century. Social planning councils, community chests, and other bodies looked to service coordination as a means of effective resource allocation. Child guidance clinics tested the use of multidisciplinary case coordination teams. Worker's compensation programs in the 1940s used a case coordination approach in their rehabilitation efforts (Kaplan, 1990). Multiservice centers for veterans returning from World War II incorporated staff from private and public provider agencies, and in the 1950s the "multiproblem family" was identified as in need of a coordinated treatment approach (Weil & Karls, 1985).

Throughout this time, case management remained largely an informal or indirect practice, delivered as part of other services and receiving little public notice. Then came the explosion of categorical social and medical programs beginning with the Great Society policies of the early 1960s, and service system fragmentation became targeted as a major problem with a new sense of urgency. This led directly to development of case management as a formal practice and distinct service.

The Categorical Imperative and the Case Management Fix

Beginning in the early 1960s, the federal government greatly expanded its commitment to human services, as well as its intervention and investment in their funding and operation. One main form of this involvement consisted of categorical programs providing resources for the provision of specialized services (such as community mental health centers) to meet the needs of special groups (such as the mentally ill or mentally retarded). Under Lyndon Johnson, Congress mandated roughly 240 categorical programs; the number continued to grow under Nixon and Ford, so that about five hundred such programs were in existence by 1980 (TenHoor, 1982). Entitlement programs were another expression of public commitment to human service systems beginning under Great Society policies, with Medicare, Medicaid, the Older Americans Act, and Aid to Families with Dependent Children all enacted by the late 1960s.

The rapid proliferation of programs and funding sources created service delivery systems that appeared anything but systematic. Fragmentation was evident at several levels: in the dispersion of responsibility for different service systems (such as health care, mental health, and social services) among separate federal and state governmental departments; in the separate organizational structures, regulations, and recording systems that accompanied that dispersion; or in the dissimilar target populations of related services within the same local communities (Hokenstad, 1982). For service agencies and providers, this fragmentation meant having to assemble programs out of disparate funding streams and regulatory mandates, each potentially with different operational standards and reporting requirements. For service recipients, it meant a bewildering maze of programs and providers, eligibility requirements, and entitlement procedures.

Critics also saw fragmentation as closely tied to other problems with service systems. Barriers to accessible care resulted from insufficient knowledge about services and from bureaucratic red tape and rigidity. Lack of continuity in the service provider or across service episodes diminished the effectiveness and quality of care. Duplication of service programs or, conversely, gaps in the care network and administrative waste all contributed to systems' ineffectiveness and inefficiency (Hokenstad, 1982).

The programs that would promote case management grew from attempts to counteract these systemic woes. The policies creating those programs did not, however, emerge in a straightforward manner from a simple recognition of the problems created by service fragmentation. To some extent, such problems had already been identified in the very legislation promoting categorical programs. The Older Americans Act of 1965, for example, emphasized the creation of comprehensive service systems at state and local levels through planning, service coordination, and resource pooling (Estes, 1979); community mental health center and comprehensive health planning legislation shared this emphasis. These measures lacked explicit definition of pooling, planning, and coordination mechanisms, and further lacked authority to mandate stronger or broader changes in the structure of service systems. They did, nonetheless, set the stage for a human service policy agenda defining the problem as one of fragmentation, with the solution being grounded in consolidation and coordination.

That agenda became a cornerstone of the "new federalism" policies of Republican administrations in the early to mid-1970s. Block grants were the most visible antithesis to the categorical program approach, since they combined disparate programs and transferred federal funds to state and local governments rather than program providers. States and communities then determined how resources would be allocated to specific program areas, given a broad latitude of goals within the federal framework. In the process, block granting widened policy objectives beyond the protection of special interests (and their administrative and organizational constituencies) and decreased the accountability and program quality demands on state and local governments that had accompanied categorical programs. Advocates also used the potential cost savings of program consolidation and simplification to justify budgetary reductions (TenHoor, 1982).

Thus, modern manifestations of case management arose not simply as a response to service system fragmentation. Case management programs developed in the 1970s within a context of attempts to realign the balance of power in the government and reduce overall public expenditures through consolidated service resources. One of the earliest revenue sources for case management programs was the social service block grant contained in Title XX of the Social Security Act, enacted in 1974. Case management was designated as one of the services for which Title XX paid, and by 1978 it was the fifteenth largest service funded under the program (TenHoor, 1982).

Title XX has all the hallmarks of the block grant model. It has a flexible approach to service goals, which are defined in five broad areas: promoting "economic self-support"; promoting "personal and social self-sufficiency"; providing community- or home-based care alternatives to institutionalization; providing institutional care when most appropriate; and prevention of abuse or neglect of children and adults, together with strengthening of the family. States could deliver any services believed appropriate to those goals, in any combination, within and across local districts. Few federal restrictions guided this decision making, save the requirement that funds had to be targeted to the poor or "medically needy" (TenHoor, 1982, p. 37). Title XX also represented a response to concerns about federal outlays for social welfare funding. A growth of 500 percent in state claims for federal matching of Social Security social service dollars between 1967 and 1972 prompted Congress to put a ceiling on such authorizations, and Title XX was capped in like manner from the beginning.

Under Title XX, case management translated the political philosophy and agenda of new federalism into policy and practice objectives of integrated, flexible care planning designed to constrain service expenditures and to enhance state, local, and organizational discretion in resource allocation. This was true as well in its other early federally sponsored manifestations, especially those that emerged under the "human services integration movement" of the late 1960s and early 1970s. Led in part by state welfare administrators who wanted to rationalize and decentralize control over service systems, the movement spawned federal sponsorship of demonstration projects with case management as service linkage components, among them the Services Integration Targets for Opportunity (SITO) program and Comprehensive Services Delivery project (TenHoor, 1982; Kaplan, 1990).

Chapters 2, 3, and 4 will demonstrate that similar policy contexts surrounded the early demonstrations of case management in the fields of long-term care, mental health, and social welfare. These early forms of case management mirrored the trends in the sectors in which they arose. These sectors were undergoing their own revolutionary changes in organization and philosophy in the early 1970s: long-term care and mental health toward deinstitutionalized, community-based care, welfare toward employment and training programs. Such movements provided rationalizing discourses that linked the objectives, assumptions, and beliefs in the sector to broader policy interests. For example, the goals of community-based care for so-called frail elders included preventing inappropriate institutionalization and delaying the need for institutional care through comprehensive service provision—goals that dovetailed nicely with arguments for cost control, decentralized authority, flexible resource allocation, and service integration strategies. Case management provided categorical programs with a relatively low cost way to demonstrate the connections between their particular goals and broader social objectives at a time when the overall policy climate was working against categorical approaches.

While the overall aims of particular case management programs might fit well with those framed at a national level, accomplishing those objectives would require operational measures that might be at odds with broader goals. For example, increasing access to services could threaten to increase overall service expenditures; or, making authority over services more decentralized could result in case management programs needing stronger procedures for advocacy, which in turn might conflict with goals of increasing interagency cooperation. As later chapters show, the tensions accruing from such contradictory objectives have played a vital role in shaping the structure of case management programs and the way case management is practiced in particular service sectors.

New Players and Payers

Since the demonstrations of the 1970s, case management has spread across a wide sweep of service sectors, propelled in part by legislative mandate. Figure 2 summarizes major federal initiatives making case management either an optional or a required part of services for populations as diverse as the developmentally disabled, the chronically mentally ill, and children in foster care. States' actions further developed the reach of case management approaches, particularly in welfare and Medicaid programs. Foundation support reinforced these public initiatives, leading to new arenas and types of case management practice; an example is the Robert Wood Johnson Foundation's Hospital Initiatives in Long-Term Care program, which prompted hospital-based models of aftercare management and community care coordination (Applebaum & Austin, 1990).

Case management now appears in an array of service settings including primary care physicians' offices, acute care hospitals, regional health care systems, programs for the homeless, clinics for high-risk pregnant women, substance abuse treatment programs, HIV risk reduction projects, lifetime care programs for persons with spinal cord injury, school-based services for teenage parents, and military family advocacy units (Ciosci & Goodman, 1994; Cohen & Cesta, 1994; Czerenda & Best, 1994; Davis, 1992; Gemmill, Kennedy, Larison, Mollerstrom, & Brubeck, 1992; Hurley & Fennell, 1990; Netting, Warrick, Christianson, & Williams, 1994; Siegal, 1994; White, Gundrum, Shearer, & Simmons, 1994). The most notable recent applications of case management are not in new sectors, however, but by new providers and payers. Beginning in the 1980s, case management became a core technology of managed health and mental health care, in traditional health maintenance organization (HMO) settings, in Social/HMOs serving older clients, and in both self-insured and third-party insurance programs. Most major insurance companies now operate with in-house or contracted case management components. Initially focused primarily on high-cost patients, the objectives of managed care case management have since broadened to wider attempts to rationalize use and contain costs incurred by subscribers as a whole (Austin, 1990; Austin & O'Connor, 1989; Hurley & Fennell, 1990; Vourlekis, 1992).

Another noteworthy innovation is that of private practice case management. Performed mainly by social workers, fee-for-service case management providing case coordination and monitoring has become a popular resource for elders and their families as well as parents with mentally disabled children (Vourlekis, 1992). This has become a sufficiently large enterprise to warrant the development of professional associations for private case managers. Allied with private practice in market orientation (if not necessarily in service goals or populations) are case manage-

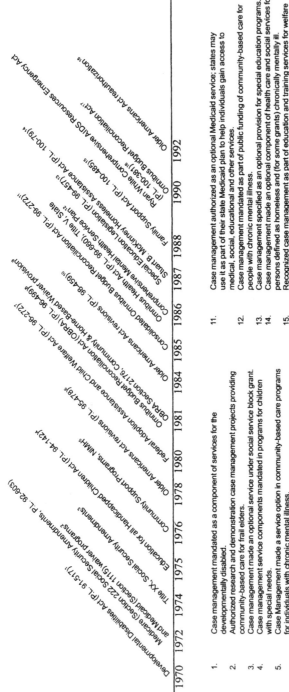

Timeline years: 1970 · 1972 · 1974 · 1975 · 1976 · 1978 · 1980 · 1981 · 1984 · 1985 · 1986 · 1987 · 1988 · 1990 · 1992

Legislation labels along the timeline:

- Developmental Disabilities Act (P.L. 91-517)[1]
- Medicare (Section 222 Social Security Amendments, P.L. 92-603)
- Title XX, Social Security Amendments[2]
- Education for all Handicapped Children Act[3]
- Community Support Programs, NIMH[4]
- Older Americans Act revisions (P.L. 94-142)[5]
- Federal Adoption Assistance and Child Welfare Act (P.L. 96-272)[7]
- OBRA Section 2176, Community & Home-Based Waiver provisions[9]
- Omnibus Budget Reconciliation Act (OBRA) (P.L. 96-499)[8]
- Older Americans Act revisions (P.L. 95-478)[6]
- Consolidated Omnibus Budget Reconciliation Act revisions (P.L. 98-459)[10]
- Comprehensive Mental Health Legislation (P.L. 99-660), Title V, State Comprehensive Mental Health Service Plan[12]
- Special Education Legislation (P.L. 99-457)[13]
- Stuart B. McKinney Homeless Assistance Act (P.L. 100-77)[14]
- Family Support Act (P.L. 100-485)[15]
- Ryan White Comprehensive AIDS Resources Emergency Act[17]
- Omnibus Budget Reconciliation Act (P.L. 100-79)[16]
- Older Americans Act reauthorization[18]

Legend:

1. Case management mandated as a component of services for the developmentally disabled.
2. Authorized research and demonstration case management projects providing community-based care for frail elders.
3. Case management made an optional service under social service block grant.
4. Case management service components mandated in programs for children with special needs.
5. Case Management made a service option in community-based care programs for individuals with chronic mental illness.
6. Case management mandated in social services for the elderly.
7. Case planning and review required in services for children in foster care.
8. Established a waiver program for primary care case management in state Medicaid plans.
9. Permitted states to develop case managed community-based care programs for Medicaid recipients at risk of nursing home institutionalization.
10. Assigned responsibility for case management programs to Area Agencies on Aging.
11. Case management authorized as an optional Medicaid service; states may use it as part of their state Medicaid plan to help individuals gain access to medical, social, educational and other services.
12. Case management mandated as part of public funding of community-based care for people with chronic mental illness.
13. Case management specified as an optional provision for special education programs.
14. Case management made an optional component of health care and social services for persons defined as homeless and (for some grants) chronically mentally ill.
15. Recognized case management as part of education and training services for welfare recipients. Permitted state agencies to require assignment of a case manager to families in jobs and training programs.
16. Case management specified as an optional component of three major service initiatives for people with HIV/AIDS.
17. Specified non-provider-based case management as an optional Medicaid service.
18. Listed independent case management as a direct service eligible for funding.

(Sources: Applebaum & Austin, 1990; Geron & Chassler, 1994; Kaplan, 1990; TenHoor, 1982; Vourlekis, 1992)

Figure 2. Case Management's Mandate: A Timeline of Federal Legislation

ment programs in Employee Assistance Programs as well as case management performed by private firms for public agencies, such as welfare and child welfare departments (Doolittle & Riccio, 1992; Hegar, 1992; N. Miller, 1992).

As described in Chapter 5, these new applications continue to face the structural, programmatic, and philosophic issues that have been inherent in case management programs from their beginning. At the same time, new case management programs confront the particular expectations and constraints attached to their service systems as well as the unique constellations of need among their clientele. This, then, yields case management practice that is protean and dynamic, even as it searches for stability and standards.

Variations on the Theme: Case Management Today

Case management today has a variety of faces. Designated case managers include physicians, nurses, social workers, psychologists, and administrative personnel with baccalaureate-level education. They may operate individually or as part of interdisciplinary teams. Case managers may see their clients in person on a daily basis, every six months, or never, for those whose contact is over the telephone. They may be specialists who process large batches of cases for a particular service, or generalists who attempt to address all the service needs of a small caseload. Case management programs may have the ability to authorize services and monitor overall expenditures, and some even assume financial risk through capped and capitated funding; others act as service brokers, securing care for clients through informal working relationships with other provider agencies.

There have been numerous attempts to understand these different types of case management on a conceptual as well as empirical level; that is, to develop typologies capturing the significant dimensions along which case management programs vary, and to evaluate which of these differences *make* a difference to program outcomes. Major instances of these evaluations are reviewed in the chapters on long-term care, mental health, and welfare, and Chapter 5 reviews current models of case management used within the United States as well as internationally. In general, we know more about *how* case management varies among sectors and programs than why. The development of these diverse forms and structures is itself generally treated as taken-for-granted history, without examining the processes generating such diversity both within and across service sectors. There has been little documentation about how case management programs respond to the different contexts in which they are located—that is, their local communities and administrative sites. Moreover, how all these sources of variation might affect client outcomes is virtually terra incognita.

One of the problems in attempting to explore such terrain has been the absence of theoretical maps and guideposts. For though the development of case management proceeded in line with theoretical advances in administrative science and the caring disciplines, those advances did more to justify the policies creating case management than to mold the research evaluating it. Such evaluation primarily has reflected administrative concerns with issues of design, efficacy, efficiency, and costs. Yet those concerns themselves have been malleable, giving priority to different issues at different times, in line with diverse policy and programmatic climates. The orienting and generalizing power of a theoretical approach has thus largely been lacking in the analysis of case management programs. The final section describes how social theory will be used in this book to shed new light on some old and new issues in the policy formulation, program design, and practice of case management.

RETHINKING CASE MANAGEMENT

This book provides a comparative analysis of case management in a variety of service settings and a critical assessment of case management as a social product and a social process. As noted earlier, this goes beyond the main body of work on the subject, which consists of practice manuals, outcome evaluations, and other analyses focused on particular programs or service sectors. The difference here is more than substantive. It involves treating as problematic that which typically has been taken for granted: the reasons for case management's existence and expansion, the sources as well as significance of its variability, and the meaning of current trends in its design and objectives. Viewing case management in this way requires new ways of thinking about what it is and what it does.

Three themes that appear in the chapters to come represent separate but related views of case management. The first examines case management as a role set at the boundary between service agencies and other organizations and providers. This boundary-spanning position fundamentally shapes the structure and practice of case management. The second theme depicts case management as an institutionalized practice; that is, a set of procedures grounded in a system of social and material relations among actors and organizations. These relations are institutionalized in two senses: They have become widely accepted and disseminated, due in part to regulatory mandate; and they are closely tied to other institutional structures in our society, including the state, the market, and race, class, and gender. The third theme is that case management represents a system of symbolic relations, in addition to its social and material ones: It is itself a concept linked to the other concepts, paradigms, and ideologies that form and shape service systems.

These views of case management draw from social constructionism, political economic perspectives, and institutional organizational theory. Though not contradictory when applied to the study of social policy, each focuses on different aspects and makes a distinctive contribution to understanding case management.

Social Constructionism

Social constructionism asserts that reality is socially constructed, generated and sustained by a collectively shared body of knowledge that exists and operates at a taken-for-granted level. Social knowledge, in this view, is the product of power relations, connected to dominant ideologies and paradigms themselves crafted in particular social and historical contexts. Though linked in that way to the status quo, social knowledge is also malleable and contestable, subject to the interaction of multiple interests and sites of power (Lupton, 1994). Social constructionism does not necessarily deny that there are phenomena (states, structural conditions, or experiences) that are "objectively real, regardless of how they are perceived," but rather takes as its focus the "socially constructed ideas that define and provide images of these phenomena," since these ideas provide the basis for social action (Estes, 1979, p. 14).

Applied to the analysis of social policy, this perspective informs us that perceptions of social problems and proposed solutions are socially constructed, negotiated in specific social and historical contexts. Because these constructions shape the way people perceive reality, they come also to assume an objective reality as they are converted into program designs and policy prescriptions: "the perceptions of what is possible become what is real" (Estes, 1979, p. 4).

We have already seen this process at work in the way social service coordination emerged from the mechanistic model of service systems to become both a perennial policy objective and a paradigm guiding the development of case management programs. Chapters 2 through 4 will examine how the paradigm of service coordination has been expressed as part of the broader policy agenda in specific service sectors, in turn shaping the conception as well as the practice of case management in different ways. Looking across various service sectors and new case management applications in Chapters 5 and 6 will further inform our understanding of the concept of case management and how it is part of broader symbolic meanings and cultural practices attached to service systems and their clients.

Political Economic Perspective

While social constructionism alerts us to the importance of symbolic elements and sociohistorical contexts, the political economic perspective points more directly to the role of the state and political and economic trends in shaping social programs and policy. This approach underscores how inequities in control over material and social resources produce differential states of health and well-being within society. Groups (such as the ill, disabled, aged, unemployed, and minorities) that do not contribute to the capitalist economy are disadvantaged and marginalized, limited in their access to the goods and services that could ameliorate their condition. Service systems, including medicine, social welfare, and social services, are such goods and services, and their distribution mirrors broader social inequalities. At the same time, such systems act as instruments of social control and reinforce the capitalist system of production in several ways: by defining need in ways that obscure its broader social structural origins, by targeting resources to those most likely to rejoin the labor market, and by promoting "the consumption of commodities to secure the healing process" (Lupton, 1994, p. 9).

Adopting a political economic perspective will help us assess the historical and political contingencies shaping the development of case management programs within service sectors. In particular, this perspective encourages analysis of how case management policy and programs respond to those environmental elements on which they depend for resources, such as funding or clients (Albrecht & Peters, 1995). On a broader level, the perspective requires that we examine how the social and material relations embedded in case management programs reflect the institutionalized social order, and specifically structures of class, race, and gender. This leads us to ask how case management systems reinforce structures of inequality even as they may seek to redress them.

We focus more directly on the role played by the state, market forces, and professional interests in the expansion of case management in Chapter 5. There and in Chapter 6 we also examine how case management programs and practitioners act as agents of social control: through the frameworks guiding the definition of need; the targeting of service resources; and relationships to service industries such as home care, rehabilitation, and employment training. This analysis helps explain the sources of case management's continued popularity and diverse applications, but also provides ways of rethinking how case management can best contribute to service system reform, as discussed in the final chapter.

Institutional Theory

The final theoretical strand woven through the book comes from theory on organizations and their environments. Despite the physical walls and institutional structures that may enclose them, organizations are open systems, responsive to demands, incentives, and opportunities present in their environments (Scott, 1981). Local environments encompass the neighboring community of other organizations or service providers, suppliers and consumers, and local political and governmental bodies; more distal environments stretch through hierarchies of funding and regulatory agents and through related sectors, industries, and markets (Scott & Meyer, 1991).

Organizations respond to both types of environments as they imprint historical developments into their structures and missions and actively strive to achieve the relationships with other environmental players that will ensure their survival (Scott, 1981). Some of the environmental challenges they face are technical in nature, related to the goods or services they produce, their amount and distribution, and the effectiveness and efficiency of production techniques. Yet other demands are related to the externally defined rules and normative requirements with which the organization must conform in order to gain support from other players in their environments. These are termed the *institutional environment* because they elaborate norms, ideologies, roles, or beliefs that act independently of technical and market requirements and that often become codified in professional and licensing rules and standards (Meyer & Rowan, 1977).

In order to survive, then, organizations must achieve not only technical viability but also normative legitimacy. One way they do this is by adjusting their structure and operations to forms considered right, appropriate, and of high caliber within their domains as well as forms of proven technical superiority. To do this requires organizations to read the trends and forces active in their environments, to monitor their connections with those forces, and to represent themselves to other players. Boundary-spanning mechanisms, such as acquisitions, public relations, marketing, and sales divisions, provide one way of accomplishing those functions (Aldrich & Herker, 1977; Adams, 1976).

Though they clearly can be useful in monitoring the technical demands of the environment, boundary-spanning mechanisms are particularly important in helping the organization respond to the institutional environment to ensure its prestige, support, and legitimacy. They establish roles for personnel (the "boundary-spanners" themselves) who have more leeway in adjusting to environmental norms and specifications than that held by core administrative or production offices; this decoupling allows the organization to preserve some autonomy at its core while also conforming to external agencies' conventions (Meyer, Scott, & Deal, 1981). In addition, boundary-spanners can use their working relations with other organizations to establish the climate of cooperation and good will thought essential to the development of mutual trust and legitimation (Meyer & Rowan, 1977).

Since a major function of case management is to link clients with needed services and to monitor those linkages, case managers become by definition boundary-spanners (though the location and permeability of the boundaries being spanned varies among programs and across sectors). The boundary-spanning nature of the role leads to differences in case management practice: "Because the case management role is necessarily diffuse and influenced by structural constraints, client contingencies, and case manager preferences, there is likely to be a great deal of variation in role performance. . . . What case managers do will be tuned to the actions and reactions of such reciprocal roles as client, client's family, service system administrator, and organization director" (Fiorentine & Grusky, 1990, pp. 80–81). In addition, the more that case managers deal with services provided by organizations other than their own, the greater the opportunity for the normative requirements, procedures, and objectives of other organizations to influence case management operations. Case management programs may then respond to local environmental differences by developing diverse operational styles and criteria of perceived effectiveness (Dill, 1994).

The concepts of institutional environment and boundary-spanning role are useful in examining the mediation of case management in different service sectors—that is, how the design and operations of case management programs respond to the demands and contingencies of their environments. Chapters 2 through 5 demonstrate that, while it may not always be so flexible as the term *organizational Rorschach* suggests, what case management is and what the case managers do in practice are both contextually defined. The possibilities and limits in case management's future will similarly depend on the broader contexts defining it.

SUMMARY AND CONCLUSION

This chapter has reviewed the definition and history of case management as a means of coordinating services for individuals with long-term, multiple needs. We have seen that case management arose as part of a policy paradigm focused on issues of organization, coordination, and productivity, attempting to remedy those problems in large part through programs directed at individual clients. This focus introduces multiple, sometimes contradictory objectives into the design and practice of case management. Case management has also been malleable in response to political dynamics and the diverse constituencies with interests in its outcomes.

Most accounts of the reasons for case management's emergence have emphasized the critical need for service coordination in response to the fragmentation, inefficiency, and confusion left in the wake of the explosion of service systems in the 1960s. We have augmented that account by noting how case management formed as part of broader attempts to realign the balance of power between federal and state levels and to reduce overall public expenditures through block granting. Subsequent chapters will show how these efforts expressed themselves in specific service sectors, and how those sectors used case management in response to their own organizational and philosophical revolutions.

In sketching out the diverse array of sites, shapes, and services that constitute case management today, we found few analytic guideposts to help explain either the expansion or the variability of the practice. This leads to three theoretically grounded views of case management: as a boundary-spanning position, as an institutionalized practice, and as a concept within a system of symbolic relations. Taken together, these theoretical perspectives will illuminate the connections between the social and historical forces producing case management programs, the structure and organization of those programs, and the nature of case management practice. Using social constructionist and political economic frameworks will help reveal the imprint of the symbolic systems (ideologies, norms, discourses, and paradigms) shaping case management operations and objectives, as well as the influence of political climates, economic trends, and institutional elements embedded in the social structure. Institutional theory will be useful in identifying the impact of the environments in which specific programs operate, and with the concept of boundary-spanning can suggest causes for differences found among case management programs and practitioners.

In an era straining for revision and control of the missions, means, and ends of human services, it is critical that we understand the meaning, as well as substance, of our policy instruments. This book seeks to add to that understanding by examining the history, concept, and practice of case management in relation to broader paradigms and prospects for service system reform.

2

Long-Term Care
for the Elderly
Case Management as Black Box and Social Movement

In the early 1970s, case management programs serving older adults operated in a few sites around the country, running as time-limited demonstration projects with public funding. Though they differed in structure, setting, and operations, these programs served a common agenda: to increase older people's use of home- and community-based services in a way that would prevent or retard their need for nursing home care. At this writing, early in the 21st century, older Americans are likely to encounter a case manager in almost any care setting they enter. The most widespread programs operate with Medicaid and Older Americans Act funding, but others draw from private as well as public sources to support case management in hospitals, hospice care, protective services, respite programs, managed care organizations, and third-party insurance systems. While their objectives are as varied as their organizational settings, these case management programs have changed from their predecessors, focusing primarily on case management's potential to control the costs of care.

This chapter examines the origins, development, and practice of case management programs serving the elderly. The emphasis is on programs providing community-based long-term care services because that has been, and continues to be, the main arena in which case management operates; that is, much of the history of case management here is also the history of home- and community-based care for older persons.[1] The first section assesses major trends and cultural currents that converged in the appearance of the early case management demonstrations, shaping as well later applications. Next, we see how case management spread into a variety of program initiatives and service settings. One major theme here is how case management retained its legitimacy despite being treated as a "black box" in program operations—that is, a form of technology which processed inputs into outputs in ways that were not well studied or understood. Indeed, case management's legitimacy as a service technology endured despite an absence of evidence that it was even effective in achieving program goals. To understand how this occurred will require examining how particular organizational and professional interests promoted case management's expansion through a social movement fostering community-based care. These themes then set the basis for the final section, when we look at particular case management programs in practice to see how their roots shape both their potential and their limitations.

BACKGROUND: THE AGING ENTERPRISE AND THE UNRIVALED MINORITY

The beginnings of formal case management programs serving older people date to a period from the mid-1960s until the end of the 1970s.[2] Legislative acts authorizing public support for services for older people set the boundaries of this period—at its outset, the enactment of Medicare, Medicaid, and the Older Americans Act, and at its end, the 1978 Older Americans Act Amendments and the 1981 Omnibus Budget Reconciliation Act. The early acts marked the zenith of Great Society efforts to expand access to health care and social services; the latter ones set the tone for a rationalization and retrenchment of service systems that have continued to this day.

That elders were seen as having problems that could and should be addressed through public action on behalf of the group as a whole was a remarkable, almost unprecedented policy stance, leading one analyst to pronounce them an "unrivaled minority" (Pratt, 1976, p. 83). While this position enjoyed broad popular support, it was also actively promoted by an array of organizations, agencies, and professional interests in governmental, corporate, nonprofit, and academic arenas. In turn, public legitimation and funding fueled the expansion of programs offered by those promoters and their consolidation as an "aging enterprise" (Estes, 1979). To understand the wellspring as well as the impact of these social images of the elderly and that of the aging enterprise, we need first to look at the demographic and political economic context of the time.

Amid the social turmoil of the 1960s, changes in the fundamental social institutions of the family and the state altered the roles of each as well as the relationship between them. Postwar economic and baby booms had prompted two decades of geographic and social mobility reinforcing the separation and significance of the nuclear family. But then the increased entry of women into the paid labor force, the rising rate of divorce, and a drop-off in the birthrate began to challenge both the dynamics and the structure of family life (Torres-Gil, 1992). With Great Society initiatives directed at such areas as employment, housing, early childhood education, and care for the aged, the role of the state expanded to formerly private domains—to support families, according to proponents, or to supplant or control them, as detractors feared.

As the administrative and policy climate changed, the "new federalism" again renegotiated the public role. Nowhere was this more clear than in health care policy, where the earlier emphasis on increasing access and the availability of care was supplanted by attempts to rationalize services and contain their costs (Brown, 1988). We find here, for instance, the first public promotion of HMOs as well as state-level experiments that would ultimately yield the change in Medicare reimbursement under the Prospective Payment System. On a broader level, and particularly following the 1976 oil crisis and the economic "stagflation" that followed, the will to expand the creation of new governmental programs eroded steadily from here on. To the extent that new services evolved, they appeared at the state or local level or, more prevalently, in the private and nonprofit sectors (Smith & Lipsky, 1993). Suspicions that families were allowing the government to take over their duties joined these trends to promote the return to the family, or "informalization," of the charge and costs of care through reins placed on public spending (Estes, Swan, & Associates, 1993).

One observer sums up the changes of these times as a refashioning of the paradigm that had shaped social welfare since the New Deal:

> That paradigm included the belief that: a succession of group-identified needs warrants government action, action is benign and helpful, family life is enhanced by relief of onerous caretaking tasks, [and] large-scale organization is efficient and responsive to human needs. . . . [In] the new one . . . government effort to improve the quality of life, in social terms, is undesirable and not benign. Families should not be so substantially relieved of traditional caring tasks as in the past. Decision making and organization should be decentralized. (Morris, 1981, p. ix)

Throughout this time, the elderly retained the aura of "deservingness" that had garnered them preferential treatment in public policy since the English Poor Laws (Rochefort, 1986). Other social images of aging and the elderly were being transformed, however. In part this reflected a different type of elderly person in a different social world. For the first time in history, a substantial proportion of the population was living into "real old age," generally in a state of reasonably good health (Morris, op. cit.), and the impact of an aging population was being foreseen. Changes in family life meant that it could not be assumed that the elderly in need of care would receive it from family members; and it was neither assumed nor desired that such care would be provided in a relative's home. Older persons were also more able to sustain their economic independence, as the first cohorts with widespread support under Social Security came of age. This meant, as well, that fewer elders remained in the paid labor force than before; those who did were polarized between those who lacked an economic alternative (disproportionately people of color and lower classes) and those able to hold onto positions of power.

Not surprisingly, polls evaluating public perceptions of aging and the elderly began to find a more positive image than had existed only shortly before.[3] This more positive view found reinforcement in the burgeoning new field of social gerontology. While in the 1950s gerontologists sought to demonstrate the mutual disengagement of elders and society from each other (a process thought inevitable and normal), emphasis in the 1960s shifted to the unused potential of older persons and the need for them to remain active and socially engaged (Rochefort, 1986). In this view, dependency was at the root of the problems of aging; the solution was thus to enhance the physical, economic, and social psychological independence of the elderly individual (Estes, 1979). Despite notice from critics that this dependency was itself grounded in social structural arrangements that promoted inequality and enforced retirement, the definition of aging in terms of individual functioning would dominate policy discussions from here on.

This definition well suited the growing ranks of professions claiming the needs of elders as their domain. Medical, public health, and social service providers, related industries, public bureaucracies at all levels, interest groups, academics and research institutes, trade associations, and individual professions—together these all constituted an aging enterprise (Estes, 1979, p. 2), a mass (though hardly unified) effort to define and treat the problems and needs of the aged. One of their first collective mobilizations came in the White House Conference on Aging in 1961, in which recommendations set the stage for policy discussions of expanded health insurance coverage of the aged (which would shortly lead to Medicare and Medicaid), as well as expansion of nursing home and home care services. The latter industries would play major roles in subsequent conferences and policy debates, affirming their place at the core of the enterprise.

Another major boost for aging services came in 1965 with the enactment of the Older Americans Act (OAA). This promoted a series of broad, universal objectives to enhance the physical, mental, social, and economic well-being of all elders and assigned the work required to achieve those objectives to health and social service providers. State-level "agencies on aging" were charged with planning, coordinating, and developing services in this system. Services funded through grants and contracts under OAA auspices would include transportation, information and referral, nutrition and meals programs, and home care and community-based care demonstrations. In most cases, the providers were local, nonprofit multipurpose social service agencies, who, with their public counterparts, thus became increasingly invested in elder care.

Over the course of the 1960s and 1970s, there were two main policy directions in long-term care. The first can be termed a "planning and coordination" service strategy (Estes, 1979). Elaborating the indirect approach to system reform adopted by the OAA from the beginning, this strategy now fell in line with the new federalism emphasis on decentralization of publicly sponsored services. In 1973, OAA amendments created local-level Area Agencies on Aging (AAAs) with a broad mandate to plan and coordinate services for the aged in their areas. Lacking any authority to enforce service plans or coordinating mechanisms, AAAs relied mainly on such strategies as encouraging communication, service integration, and joint ventures among local providers. Both fostering and complicating such strategies were the limited funding available for direct services and the introduction at this time of block grants replacing formerly categorical program grants for social services and community development. Service agencies thus increasingly jostled, competed, and collaborated in the quest for funding.

The 1978 reauthorization of the OAA again emphasized that the problems of the aged were appropriately addressed by continued attention to planning and coordination. This framing clearly responded to the pressures of what was by now commonly called an "aging network" of service providers and public agencies (Gelfand, Olsen, & Berman, 1980), who were major figures in the reauthorization hearings.[4] Area agencies now received more discretionary authority in determining which needs of elders should have priority in their community; they were also encouraged to "designate, wherever feasible, a focal point agency for the delivery of comprehensive coordinated services within the community" (Estes, 1979, p. 46). A separate provision created the authority to fund these focal point community-based care programs as model projects to "provide for identification and assessment of long-term care needs of individual elderly persons, referral of such persons to the appropriate services, follow-up and evaluation of the continued appropriateness of such services" (Congressional Record, 1978, p. S11538, cited in Estes, 1979, p. 48). This, then, became a source of support for the earliest case management programs.

Accompanying the coordination approach by the late 1960s was a second policy direction—a widespread push at state and local levels to expand community-based services for the elderly. There had already been an explosion of community resources for older people, including nutritional, transportation, informational, housing-related, and home care services. What proponents put forward now was that these services still were not reaching enough people, and that extending their reach would enable the elderly to avoid having to enter an institution.

Paralleling deinstitutionalization within mental health, this movement garnered support from many sources. Those representing social service and health care agencies pointed to research indicating that as many as 15 to 30% of nursing home residents were there not because of a need for nursing care, but because of a lack of alternative services in the community (Sherwood, 1975; Bell, 1973; Pfeiffer, 1973). Further reinforcing their case were media exposés of abusive conditions in nursing homes as well as studies indicating high levels of unmet home health needs among elders in the community (Kahana & Coe, 1975; Benjamin, 1993).

In addition to service agencies, professional interests played an expansionary role. The American Nurses Association, the American Medical Association (AMA), and organizations representing voluntary social service agencies had supported home care as a way to control hospital spending even before the enactment of Medicaid and Medicare (Benjamin, 1993). Public health nursing had remained particularly critical of the limitations in long-term care coverage under those programs, and particularly the dominance of medicine in determining the scope of care (Mundinger, 1983). Fueling the concern of social work organizations at this time were aspersions on the efficacy of casework made by the federal administration as well as from within the profession (see review by Fischer, 1973). Community-based services offered the potential to prove the worth of the social service approach.

A move away from services provided in hospitals and nursing homes was also attractive to public agencies and policymakers because of the rising costs of such care under Medicare and Medicaid reimbursement.[5] Until this point, Medicare's home health benefit was limited fiscally and restricted to a medical model of care linked to skilled nursing and directed by physicians. Medicaid allowed states greater latitude in providing a wider range of services (including more social and homemaker services) to those with chronic illness and low incomes, but in practice most states limited the availability of home health care through restrictions on benefits and reimbursement (Benjamin, 1993). Though there was widespread federal interest in expanding home- and community-based care as an alternative to nursing home care, agencies were divided regarding what types of services could be expanded, and with what level of entitlement. The Public Health Service, long a supporter of chronic care, now boosted expansion of home health care, including homemaker services. Allied with this stance was the Administration on Aging as well as congressional committees on aging, while the Social Security Agency and the Social and Rehabilitation Service, concerned about the fiscal integrity of Medicare and Medicaid, respectively, wanted any expansion to stick with a medical model of care under tight reimbursement controls (Benjamin, op. cit.).

Calls for community care expansion began to mount in such venues as state- and federal-level congressional hearings, recommendations from the U.S. General Accounting Office, professional meetings, and the 1971 White House Conference on Aging. In the latter, sessions on long-term care, physical and mental health, and homemaker-home health aide services uniformly recommended the development of "a continuum of health and social services to people in their own homes" (1971 White House Conference on Aging, p. 115) as an alternative to institutions. The push in this direction clearly came from the planning committees for these sessions, which were staffed by representatives of both public and nongovernment sectors of the aging enterprise; but widespread support by delegates at large was apparent at the Special Concerns Session on Long-Term Care as well as almost unanimous support in votes on the panels' resolutions.

Further evident at the White House Conference was a push to link community care with a policy strategy focused on coordination. This was voiced most concisely by the Delegates to the Physical and Mental Health Section in the recommendation that "A coordinated delivery system for comprehensive health services must be developed, legislated, and financed to ensure continuity of both short- and long-term care for the aged" (1971 White House Conference on Aging, p. 23). The policy emphasis had clearly shifted from program expansion to service integration. An economic context of mounting deficits, high inflation, and erratic growth joined with a political context asserting the need for rationalized, controlled care systems (Brown, 1988); these contexts would not be well inclined toward calls merely to expand community services, or to increase elders' access to them. The rhetorical tack of community care proponents was thus to acknowledge that while community services had become widespread,

> It is rare, indeed, to find in any community an adequate coordination of services and agencies involved with programs for the older population. There is too often overlapping of responsibility and authority, duplication of services, and shifting of patients from one agency to another, with fragmentation of available treatment resources, difficulty of communication at the professional level, and a sharp separation of outpatient, inpatient, and aftercare services which are not in the best interest of patients. (The Technical Committee on Physical and Mental Health, 1971 White House Conference on Aging, pp. 65–66)

The claim here was that a lack of coordination at the systems level resulted in lack of continuity and coordination in the care provided individuals. The service strategy being proposed by the early 1970s thus did not focus on the creation of new community care programs but rather the case-by-case coordination of those already there, targeting them to prevent institutionalization. Crucial to the latter was the use of a "preventive approach" using "community outreach" and "case finding" to "seek out people with medical and psychosocial needs, handling these needs early, and thus insuring continued independent living" (Kahana & Coe, 1975, p. 526). This, then, was the key that would allow service providers to expand services in the name of a coordinated approach, and it centered on identifying all elders as potentially in need of their assistance. This framing of the problem, very much in line with broader efforts at service system rationalization, would continue to dominate the policy discourse for almost two decades.

Certainly the funding and provision of services had developed in an uncoordinated manner. It was, however, supposition (supported by the anecdotal evidence of service providers themselves) that this lack of coordination translated into confusion about which services clients could get, and how. That receiving such services in a timely and coordinated manner would enable substantial numbers of elders to remain in the community was, at this point, further supposition. There was already, however, reason to doubt that such would be the case. A 4-year, randomized case-control study published in 1971 had found, for example, that elders who received comprehensive social services became increasingly dependent, ultimately experiencing higher rates of institutionalization than the control group members who received no such services (Blenkner, Bloom, & Nielson, 1971). Broader critiques of the coordination strategy noted that it could not address more fundamental needs for better incomes, health care, or housing among elders, and that there was no evidence that coordination would accomplish anything tangible in the absence of economic or political incentives (Estes, 1979).

By the early 1970s, coordinated community care was nonetheless primary on the policy agenda. The main hurdle remaining came from federal reluctance to expand Medicare and Medicaid programs to cover new services with largely unknown costs and benefits. Authorizing new programs on a demonstration basis provided the necessary compromise. As stated by one historian of the home care policy,

> Experimenting with alternatives to institutional care permitted persons who were concerned with fiscal integrity issues to examine actual programmatic experience and costs, but on a conservative scale; it gave advocates the opportunity to build their case more emphatically and concretely; and it provided time for further debate on the issues to those who were ambivalent. (Benjamin, 1993, p. 144)

The 1972 amendments to Medicare legislation provided for new experiments and demonstration programs offering services not currently covered under Medicare. This, then, initiated federal support for case managed long-term care.

The net effect of the preceding trends was that before case management programs even began, their operations were framed by a set of assumptions: that the elderly as a group both needed and deserved publicly funded assistance; that the problems of the elderly could be treated at the level of individual cases; that a major goal was to promote independent functioning in community settings; that health care and social service professionals were in the best position to assess needs and develop care plans; and that coordination of care at the case level was essential to achieve goals in a cost-effective manner. In the next section we will see how these assumptions would continue to shape case management programs through the subsequent decades—sometimes as implicit principles, other times as rhetorical statements justifying the continuation of programs that seemed not to be achieving their goals.

THE HISTORY OF CASE MANAGEMENT: A NET FOR THE AGING NETWORK

Case Management Pioneers

The first generation of community-based care programs centered on case management developed in the early to mid-1970s. Initially, these were projects sponsored through state and local service agency initiatives. Once they were able to use the projects to leverage public support, these agencies built up their program capacity and developed short-term (generally 3-year) demonstration project status, joined by new projects responding to the federal incentives. This first generation of case-managed programs grew primarily in response to the concerns reviewed previously: that care for the elderly was institutionally biased, failed to meet the needs of many who could be served in the community, and cost too much relative to its effectiveness.

Corresponding to these multiple concerns, the projects had diverse objectives aimed at different levels. At a systems level, they sought to build a safety net to support elders in their homes by expanding and coordinating the array of essential services. Such services included homemaking, transportation, adult day care, caregiver respite, and a multitude of other more social and personal care services in addition to home nursing and other medically oriented therapies. Controlling costs, of the projects themselves as well as the total service package, was a second systems-level project objective. Most early programs sought to control costs by targeting those elders who would benefit from community-based services delivered in a cost-effective manner. Only a few projects placed caps on individual client or total project expenditures, linking them to a portion of the costs of nursing home care.

Mirroring these systems-level goals, project objectives for individual clients also centered on arranging and coordinating care that incorporated "the appropriate types and levels of services in the least restrictive setting and in the most cost-effective manner" (Stassen & Holahan, 1981, p. 9). In practice, this translated into identifying clients most at risk of institutionalization, assembling a service package designed to prevent such an outcome, and adjusting the care package as needed by monitoring the client over time. These screening, packaging, and monitoring functions were precisely the domain of case management, and case managers became central to the operations of these programs.

Early community-based care projects received a major impetus from 1972 amendments to the Social Security Act that authorized the Health Care Financing Administration to fund research and demonstration projects through waivers of Medicare (Section 222 of the Social Security Amendments, P.L. 92–603) and Medicaid (Section 1115) requirements. (See Rabin & Stockton, 1986, or Zawadski, 1984a, for discussion of these different acts.)[6] Some of the best known and assessed waivered projects were the Worcester Home Care demonstration; ACCESS, the Monroe County Long-Term Care Program in New York; the Alternative Health Services (AHS) Program in Georgia; Community-Based Care Systems for the Functionally Disabled in Washington State; the Community Care Organization in Wisconsin; and Triage, Inc. in Connecticut (Kemper, Applebaum, & Harrigan, 1987; Stassen & Holahan, 1981; Weissert, Cready, & Pawelak, 1988). Case management was a mandated ingredient of each.

The design of case management reflected both local contingencies and operational philosophies. Most community care projects, for example, were created specifically for the demonstration as new programs; later projects would build exclusively on extant service provider agencies. In part, of course, this reflected an absence of programs to perform the many complex functions involved with the newly created waivered services. It also, however, bespoke the innovators' beliefs that placing case management in the hands of direct service providers would create a conflict of interest between the need for case managers to develop care plans autonomously and implicit or explicit pressures to use the services of the host agency (Applebaum & Austin, 1990).

Though controlling costs was a stated objective of these programs, case management was not primarily oriented toward direct cost constraint or gatekeeping of services. The assumption was, rather, that the appropriate and timely delivery of community-based services would save money in the end by substituting for more expensive institutional care. Both in controlling costs and in securing access, however, the programs had design limitations. Case managers had the ability to authorize services under Medicare and/or Medicaid waivers, but could only act as "brokers" for other services by making referrals to provider agencies on the client's behalf. While waivered services were often both extensive and intensive,[7] they were far from exhaustive in covering medical, economic, and social needs. Furthermore, agencies providing waivered services operated through subcontracts to demonstration programs; thus, competition for these service resources largely ceased with the signing of the contract. While projects had some financial control, their purchasing power was thus limited. Equally limited was the ability of case managers to control, or even to monitor, the total costs of care packages.

As demonstrations, these programs were required to maintain standardized records on client characteristics, administrative and service procedures, and programmatic, cost, and client outcomes. Evaluation studies, done both in-house and by independent researchers, then assessed project results, generally comparing them with data collected on a comparison group of elders in the same area who were not enrolled in the program. The initial evaluations of these early programs yielded complex and indeterminate results (Stassen & Hollahan, 1981; Weissert, 1985). While some showed reductions in nursing home use among their clients (compared to control groups), others found no difference or even higher rates of institutionalization. On most measures tracking client outcomes—from mortality to functional status or satisfaction with services—little change was evident relative to comparison groups. Moreover, there was little evidence of cost savings, with most projects, in fact, increasing total costs as they augmented the use of community-based services.

Project proponents sought to explain these generally disappointing results in two ways. The first held that methodological problems obscured the "true" program effects. For example, the reliance on comparison site data, rather than experimental, random assignment designs, meant that outcomes (whether positive or negative) would not necessarily reflect the effectiveness of the demonstration programs, since too many potentially intervening factors remained at large. The lack of comparability among programs in design and technology was another methodological issue that made generalizations across these early efforts almost impossible. Proponents thus called for more systematic, controlled comparisons using standardized program designs.

A second rationale for poor results was that programs had failed to identify and enroll the most at-risk elders, that is, those most likely to enter nursing homes. Part of the problem here was the fact that so little was known about what actually would be predictive of nursing home utilization. Absent this knowledge, it was impossible to draw a "but for" conclusion—that is, to say with certainty that clients would have entered nursing homes but for the provision of services by the program. This led programs to argue that what they needed was better means and criteria for targeting the at-risk elder.

Program operations, including case management, remained largely unexamined. Although projects kept records of case managers' activities for administrative purposes, these were rarely analyzed. Case management was thus essentially a black box: Evaluators measured project inputs (such as client characteristics and service resources) and outputs (e.g., utilization rates, costs, client outcomes) compared to those of control populations, but with little ability to examine whether results were attributable to case management (and if so, to which aspects of it) or to other programmatic elements (such as augmented service access). Such examination would have to wait until future efforts to compare projects differing in basic case management features.

A Broadening of Support

Notwithstanding the equivocal results of these early programs and the lack of understanding of exactly what they did, a new set of case management initiatives shortly followed them, beginning in the late 1970s and lasting in several cases until the present. To understand this momentum, it is necessary to examine several programmatic developments that arose around the same time as the early case management efforts and, like them, facilitated care for elders within community settings. Together, these programs raised support for the case management approach by expanding the constituency of agencies, clients and families invested in community-based care and case-level coordination strategies.

One impetus came from programs providing a greater level of home care services than that reimbursed under Medicare or Medicaid.[8] Many of these, like the community care demonstrations, drew funding from Section 222 of the 1972 Social Security Act Amendments, which waived several Medicare requirements for homemaker services. And as with the community-based care programs, the objective was to substitute in-home for institutional care and thereby to lower total long-term care expenses. Further support for home care came from federal funding for social services through matching grant funds to states under Title XX of the Social Security Act, implemented in 1975. Title XX's program goals centered on reducing institutional care by providing community-based services; the home care commonly offered by states were homemaker, chore aide, and home management services. Estimates indicated that by the early 1980s between 10 and 20% of Title XX program funds supported services for the elderly (Rabin & Stockton, 1987).

An alternate approach came in the form of experimental day care programs for older people. Section 222 funds again initiated most of these demonstrations, which were mandated to provide a variety of health and social services. These programs conducted an internal form of case management by offering so many services directly, using multidisciplinary staff for client assessments, care planning, and monitoring. As time went on, this direct service approach would evolve into a consolidated service model with the potential for fiscal accountability (Zawadski, 1984a). The main leader in this direction was the On Lok Senior Day Health Center in San Francisco, reviewed further subsequently (Ansak & Zawadski, 1984).

Yet further support for case management came at this time from the Older Americans Act (OAA). Since 1965, Title III of the act had funded a variety of home care and community-based services aimed at the elderly. Legislation reauthorizing and amending OAA in the mid-1970s further promoted the development of coordinated service systems for older persons through the Area Agencies on Aging (AAAs). AAAs were local or regional-level organizations responsible for the development of comprehensive systems centered on in-home services, overseeing the contracts or grants for direct services. In practice, this generally involved the use of case management (Rabin & Stockton, 1987; Estes, 1979).

By the early 1980s, staff and providers from the AAAs, community-based care demonstration projects, day care centers, and other home care programs had coalesced in professional networks advancing the overall goal of community care and debating their best means and practices. Different program representatives could routinely be found presenting together at professional meetings such as those of the American Public Health Association (APHA) and the Gerontological Society of America (GSA).[9] This group had major visibility at the 1981 White House Conference on Aging, where delegates overwhelmingly approved a recommendation resolving "to expand Medicare and Medicaid to provide fully for a long-term care system with case management and comprehensive in-home and out-of-home health, mental and social services . . ." (Final Report of the 1981 White House Conference on Aging, vol. 2, p. 112).[10] They had, in short, become "moral entrepreneurs" (Hasenfeld, 1992, p. 11) promoting community care as a social movement. The momentum they gained in these early days would help them keep this movement going through the rocky political times and program evaluation disappointments that lay ahead.

The Second Generation: Fiscal and Professional Control

Unlike the earliest community care demonstrations, those beginning in the late 1970s and early 1980s took place predominantly in established agencies. These included home care and other providers as well as governmental offices that had by now been involved with other home care and service coordination initiatives (Zawadski, 1984a). They thus drew on a ripening expertise in planning, grant writing, evaluation research, and consortium-building present in local service communities. In most cases, the newer community care projects grew out of pilot programs or key staff initiatives, nurtured over time by diverse funding sources and, often, state governmental sponsorship, in addition to Medicare and Medicaid waivers. At a time of increased restraint on public coffers, they also provided a way for state and local agencies to expand their domains. Some projects represented the second generation of earlier case management programs; this was the case, for example, with Triage, which began operations in 1974 with state funding and a start-up grant of OAA funds, augmenting these in 1976 with a Public Health Service research grant, and, in 1979, Health Care Financing Administration (HCFA) waivers supporting a second phase of project operations (Quinn & Hodgson, 1984).

The newer waivered programs shared the same basic orientations and objectives as the earlier ones, but with greater emphasis on targeting and cost containment. This came in the form of increased fiscal control: Several programs operated with budget limitations and caps on expenditures, while others had the authority to "pre-admission screen" all nursing home applicants seeking Medicaid benefits, rejecting such placement for those who could be served in community settings on a more cost-effective basis (Capitman, 1986; Capitman, Haskins, & Bernstein, 1986). Both budget caps and preadmission screening also tightened the targeting of services to clients, since they gave programs greater incentives and more effective mechanisms to identify and serve the at-risk population.

The emphasis on targeting and cost containment required an increased scope of managerial activities, which, in turn, translated into a more complex and professionalized system of case management than that in earlier programs (Applebaum & Austin, 1990). Projects thus tended to have higher proportions of staff with advanced training and certification. For example, none of the staff for the first phase of Triage had advanced professional training, while 75% of the staff of the program's second phase did (Capitman, 1986).

While some programs developed specialized case management functions (for example, assigning care planning to more qualified workers), more commonly used was a "casework model," with all staff members able to perform most case management activities and individual caseworkers assigned to individual clients (Capitman et al. , 1986, p. 400). Caseworkers were either more advanced in professional training or, if lower-level professionals, they worked under the guidance or supervision of more qualified professionals. The casework model thus further increased the extent to which case management was becoming a professionalized activity, though simultaneously one vulnerable to deskilling through the use of paraprofessionals.

The outcomes of these later demonstrations, like those of their predecessors, were mixed but in general disappointing to those who had hoped the improvements in program design would yield more clearly favorable results. Two separate overarching evaluations found few results of any strength (substantively or statistically) in the outcome data of these programs, and many instances in which the results of one study were contradicted by another. One of the metaevaluations found that community-based services did not, in general, reduce institutionalization or overall service costs, but did have some mild positive effects on client outcomes (Kemper et al., 1987). The absence of stronger results was a letdown, since more of these programs had randomly assigned potential clients to treatment and control groups and could thus be more confident in their findings than the comparison group evaluations of earlier programs.

The other overarching evaluation, focusing specifically on the outcomes of different case management models, found little to suggest which case management models or mechanisms were most successful, and indeed few indications of the overall effectiveness of case management per se (Capitman et al., 1986). For example, while free-standing programs with fewer professional staff and less specialization had lower case management production costs, this did not translate into lower costs for the service package overall. Resource control measures did appear to increase overall cost-effectiveness, and preadmission screening did yield reductions in nursing home use. These devices did not, however, require a case management program to support them; in fact, they could easily be utilized in programs lacking the full array of case management functions. Further, it was impossible to isolate the effects of case management or other program design elements, leading the authors to speculate "that such program features as targeting and intervention approach are at least as important in determining overall project goal attainment as are the characteristics of case management approaches" (Capitman et al., op. cit., p. 403).[11]

In all, the second set of waiver demonstration programs had again failed to satisfy their advocates' expectations. Supporters could point to various issues warranting continued program operation and further research; for example, though preadmission screening appeared to reduce nursing home use, it was unclear whether this would pertain in states with variable levels of supply and demand for nursing home and hospital beds. Advocates further pointed to the limitations that accrued from the programs' status as demonstration projects, such as the fiscal weight of start-up and research expenses, and the way 3-year time limits compromised the development of leadership and other skills within the system. Extending programs' duration and scope of operations might, it was argued, counteract these shortcomings (Zawadski, 1984b; Quinn & Hodgson, 1984).

The next stage in community-based care development centered on responses to these limitations. Two seemingly different directions would ensue. On the one hand, there was a mass diffusion of community-based care initiatives centered on case management mechanisms. For the most part, these programs emerged from services for specific population subgroups, such as Medicaid recipients. Rather than being designed to test the overall worth of community care, they represented applications of such care toward more specific ends. They would further increase the variety of case management forms and the organizational structures surrounding them. The second initiative, in contrast, was a major federal research demonstration, the Channeling project, intended to settle the lingering questions about the most effective way to structure case-managed community care.

The States Move Ahead

By the early 1980s, social policies promoted a broader conservative agenda aimed at greater state autonomy and less federal expenditure. In the human services, cost control became a paramount programmatic objective. Both the Social Services Block Grant (1981 amendments to Title XX of the Social Security Act) and the 1981 Omnibus Budget Reconciliation Act (OBRA) gave states more flexibility in the use of an increasingly limited pool of federal funds to develop community care alternatives.

Under the social service block grant program, states no longer had to provide specific services; instead, they negotiated the annual distribution of funds with local governments, which in turn determined allocations to service providers (N. A. Miller, 1992; Rabin & Stockton, 1987). As a low-cost service that did not require structural change in the overall system, case management was one of the programs typically developed. Claiming to provide case management also helped give local service agencies a competitive edge in annual appropriation decisions.

While Title XX services had limited impact because of their funding restrictions, much broader effects came from OBRA's incentives for states to expand case-managed community care programs under Medicaid through demonstration programs (under Section 2175) and the substitution of home- and community-based services for institutional care (Section 2176; Zawadski, 1984a). Unlike the earlier Medicaid 1115 demonstrations, these waivers allowed programs to run with unlimited renewals and without extensive research requirements; they also used competitive bidding among potential sites as a cost control mechanism. Services that states could offer included respite care, rehabilitation services, adult day health care, and case management, among others. Section 2176 further endowed these programs with gatekeeping and financial control measures of budget caps and preadmission screening.

States quickly took advantage of these options: By early 1983, 34 states had applied for "2176" waivers, and by the end of 1986, 41 states hosted over one hundred approved waiver programs (N. A. Miller, 1992; Applebaum & Austin, 1990). Case management was the service most commonly provided by these programs, and in 1986, a separate amendment established case management as a discrete Medicaid optional service for designated target populations. Again, states responded favorably: By 1988, 19 had approved programs for Medicaid case management, and six others awaited approval (Vourlekis, 1992). Budgetary restraints restricted the overall scope of these programs, however (Weissert, 1988).

A third funding stream diffusing case management at this time came through the Older Americans Act. In 1986, a new subsection of Title III authorized payment for a full range of nonmedical in-home services, including homemakers, friendly visiting, adult day care, and respite care. As the designated planners and coordinators of these services, Area Agencies on Aging (AAAs) relied heavily on case management, though the exact nature of case management varied from information and brokerage systems to programs acting as service gatekeepers (Applebaum & Austin, 1990). Despite the widespread nature of AAA services, funding restrictions limited their overall impact on the service system (N. A. Miller, 1992).

The significance of 2176 waiver programs and case management in AAAs transcended their funding limitations, however. Essentially, these programs institutionalized case management in diverse areas of the long-term care service community. By doing so, they legitimized it as a service technology; indeed, the legitimating process was mutual, since agencies could themselves use the inclusion of case management as a selling point for their programs. At the same time, these programs further diversified the repertoire of case management forms and functions, but still with little understanding of how differences among case management programs might result in different costs, program effects, or client outcomes.

Starting in 1981, the Department of Health and Human Services sponsored a carefully designed demonstration intended to provide definitive answers to questions about the relative effectiveness of different case management models in home and community-based care. The National Long Term Care Demonstration (commonly referred to as the Channeling Demonstration or simply Channeling) began in 1982 and ended in 1985. While largely contemporaneous with the later wave of waiver demonstration projects, it sought to correct their methodological flaws and to test critical outcome issues.

Channeling: A Definitive Test

Channeling offered several advantages for comparing different case-managed community-based care approaches (Carcagno & Kemper, 1988). It had multiple sites in 10 states throughout the country, with random as-

signment of clients at each site into program and control samples. The total sample of over 6,300 far exceeded the sizes of previous demonstrations.
Data sources available to Channeling also topped those of other programs;
beyond client interviews, program records, and Medicare and Medicaid
data, Channeling obtained information on services covered through other
means, examined death records, and interviewed clients' informal caregivers.

Channeling provided the first systematic comparison of two contrasting models of case management. One was basically a brokerage model, in
which case managers conducted needs assessments and attempted to
arrange and coordinate services to meet identified needs. In this "Basic"
approach, only a small amount of discretionary funding enabled case managers to secure any direct services. In the "Financial Control Model," on
the other hand, case managers acted as gatekeepers authorizing the
amount, extent, and duration of services under Medicare and Medicaid
waivers. They could also extend funds to purchase community services not
covered by public programs. With this largesse of resources came fiscal accountability in the form of caps on average and individual client expenditures, as well as cost sharing by higher-income clients.

The Basic and Financial Control models shared key overall objectives:
"controlling the costs of long-term care while maintaining or improving
the quality of clients' and informal caregivers' lives" (Carcagno & Kemper,
1988, p. 4). Case management activities were vital to the achievement of
these ends, and case managers in both models were expected to provide
services that were more intense, of wider scope, more integrative, and/or
of longer duration than those otherwise available in the community
(Phillips, Kemper, & Applebaum, 1988). The Channeling researchers found
in program site communities a variety of providers offering services
claimed to be "case management." Most of this, however, was care management—that is, it was connected to the provision of direct services and
thus differed in intensity, scope of services, and/or duration from the comprehensive Channeling approach. Examples included service arrangements made by hospital discharge planners and home health agencies.
About 1 in 7 individuals in the control groups of Basic model sites, and almost 1 in 5 in Financial Control sites, received more comprehensive case
management through agencies such as mental health agencies, multiservice social service agencies, and special home health care services with
pooled funding sources. These findings affirm both the diffusion of case
management activities throughout service communities at this point and
the diffuse nature of the concept of case management.

Because its evaluators looked inside the black box to discover how case
management activities might vary between the two models, Channeling
yielded a considerable amount of new information on the dynamics as well

as outcomes of case management in community-based care. First, it turned out that what case managers actually did varied in line with the structure of their programs. For example, case managers in the Basic model appeared to perform a wider array of case management activities, particularly in connection with contacts with clients and their caregivers. Financial Control case managers, in contrast, largely focused their actions around the requirements induced by the provision of formal services (Philips et al, 1988.). These differences clearly related to the control over service resources in the latter model and, in the former, a need to enhance the informal caregiving system and its link to formal services.

There was also some evidence suggesting that case managers in the two models differed in their perception of client needs. An analysis of a sample of case files revealed that, despite overall similarity in client characteristics, Financial Control case managers identified more needs related to physical and mental abilities, in response to which they secured home care and other services. Basic model case managers were more likely to identify a range of client problems related to living in the community, such as insufficient money, inadequate housing, need for legal assistance, and poor informal support. In both instances, the case managers apparently perceived client need in a way congruent with what they were able to do for the client—in the Financial Control model, through direct service provision, and in the Basic model, through case management assessment and referral.

Given that the two case management models appeared to yield different types of programs, there was surprisingly little difference in their outcomes. Most succinctly, neither seemed to make much difference for clients compared to control group members.[12] Neither significantly affected the use of nursing homes, hospitals, or other medical services, and both increased the use of community-based services, particularly personal care and homemaker services. Since program and service costs were not outweighed by lowered rates of nursing home use, both models increased the total costs of care packages.

As far as client outcomes, most measures again showed no impact by either model. This pertained to longevity as well as various quality of life indicators (such as social interaction, morale, and self-perceived health) and measures of functional health.[13]

The one area in which both models yielded benefits concerned the way clients and their caregivers responded to the services they received. By decreasing the level of clients' perceived unmet needs through increased access to care, the programs raised clients' confidence in and satisfaction with their services. The Financial Control model (which furnished significantly more services) had the same effect on caregivers' satisfaction and confidence levels, and neither program reduced the extent of informal caregiving.

Despite the care taken in planning Channeling, methodological and design issues could still have been responsible for some of these null results. For example, though apparently successful in targeting people with significant physical impairment, Channeling did not find those at high risk of nursing home use, as evidenced by findings that only 13 to 14% of the control samples entered homes after one year (Kemper, 1988). Further deflating the effects of Channeling programs may have been their deliberate location in sites already well endowed with community services.[14] Even acknowledging various factors dampening Channeling's power, it was impossible to discount the bottom line: The program did not achieve what it intended, and what it did achieve was hardly a persuasive argument for a comprehensive case-managed approach to community care. Capping two decades of demonstrations, with more than two dozen programs, yielding essentially the same null results, Channeling did in some ways provide a definitive answer to the question of whether community care could provide a cost-effective substitute to institutionalization—and the answer was "no."

The Questioned Community

Though this conclusion was no longer tentative, its broader policy significance was far from clear. Some analysts asserted that Channeling's results argued for a reevaluation of the objectives of such programs rather than further tinkering with design issues. Specifically, it seemed clear that achieving cost savings through substituting for nursing home use was no longer (if it ever had been) a valid goal for such programs, let alone a paradigm that should govern their construction (Weissert, 1988; Kane, 1988). What, then, could substitute for such substitution as a policy objective? One analyst among many rethinking such issues concluded that community-based care "has functioned primarily, and all but exclusively, as a support system for family caretakers. It is a palliative for patients not sick enough to actually enter nursing homes . . . but sick in too many ways to be helped effectively by the episodic and medically oriented health care system we have developed in this nation" (Weissert, 1988, p. 430). While this justified, to him, continuation of these programs, it also required a refocusing of their objectives, away from substituting for institutionalization and toward recognizing the programs as "a new service directed to a new population" (Ibid.), namely those persons who are functionally dependent and their caregivers.

By the time Channeling had finished, the policy environment had changed dramatically from the early days of community care demonstrations. There was even greater emphasis on cost containment, as witnessed by the inauguration of the Medicare Prospective Payment System and the Social Service Block Grants, which not only restructured but also greatly curtailed federal resource commitments (Estes et al., 1993). Given the overall political and fiscal conservatism, sponsoring community care increasingly involved a zero-sum game: If community care won, other services would suffer. Proponents thus began to argue for the importance of making sure that community-based services were equitably distributed, as well as finding ways to make them more effective and efficient (Weissert, 1988; Kane, 1988; Kemper et al., 1987; Capitman, 1986).

The call for a refocusing of community care policy was less a matter of changing objectives to fit what the programs had been able to do, than a strategy of *realpolitik*. Even as it was clear that there would no longer be public sponsorship of free-standing programs like Channeling, community-based care had become entrenched through other programs, such as the 2176 Medicaid waivers. Policy and research would henceforth focus on how to rationalize these and other systems of care and make them more productive.

Case management from here on thus became largely decoupled from the community care movement. A few case management community care demonstrations would continue, riding the waves of momentous changes in medical and long-term care from the mid-1980s on. Triage, for example, became a private agency and restructured to assume responsibility for all Medicaid and Medicare home care waiver programs in the state of Connecticut, in the process renaming itself Connecticut Continuing Care, Inc. More generally, however, the objectives of the earlier movement would be served through other programs, while case management programs would develop in an expanding array of settings.

Case Management Since the 1980s: The Contracting Regime and Corporate Profit

Over the last two decades, case management has assumed even greater variability than before, ranging from its long-standing brokerage approach to models based on standardized careplans and tight fiscal control. As a neutral technology, case management had by the mid-1980s become adaptable to almost any organizational structure and set of goals, while the functions of case managers varied depending on their fiscal control and authority over service resources.

At the same time, the multiple objectives served by case-managed community care programs have splintered into different programmatic thrusts. Goals related to the coordination of comprehensive care systems have found new expression in managed care organizations in the health care domain as well as Assisted Living and Continuing Care Retirement Communities. The goal of preventing or postponing nursing home use has largely been subsumed by constraints on the number of nursing home beds and by programs, such as respite care, hospice, and support groups, attempting to alleviate "caregiver burden" (Kane & Kane, 1987).

In part, the diffusion of case management and the splintering of community care goals have both resulted from changes in the social service and health care systems. For social services, the relationship between the nonprofit sector and the public arena has become paradoxically both strained and increasingly symbiotic over this course of time. On the one hand, block grants and other funding reductions greatly restricted the resources available within the service community, with state, private, and philanthropic contributions only partially offsetting the balance (Estes et al., 1993). Funding through the Older Americans Act, for example, declined 36% in real dollars between 1980 and 1991. Nonprofits were additionally hit by political attacks on their tax exemptions and subsidies.

At the same time, governmental agencies looked to the nonprofit arena to initiate new programs and services beyond what the conservative policy climate would support in the public domain. The contractual relations between public and nonprofit agencies that had existed since the Great Society now consolidated into a "contracting regime," in which those receiving contracts often had substantial input into the formulation, standards, and evaluation of programs (Smith & Lipsky, 1993).

Thus, social service agencies were faced with a more competitive environment, in which fewer overall resources were available. At the same time, agencies that aimed their programs in the favored directions could establish sustaining links with public funding streams. As community care became reconfigured into different types of programs for different groups in need, competitive advantages accrued to agencies that could demonstrate a track record of using accepted service technologies and approaches such as case management, even when there were fewer services to manage. Furthermore, the policy climate clearly favored such mechanisms for cost containment and system rationalization as case management and other indirect services such as assessment, information and referral, and managed care.

Changes in case management within this time span are also directly linked to a dramatic restructuring of the health care system aimed primarily at increasing the profit of medical and medically related services. Corporate entities (largely proprietary but also nonprofit) consolidated chains of the same type of providers (particularly hospitals, nursing homes, and home care agencies) in "horizontal integration" and "vertically" integrated different providers into supplier chains (Estes et al., 1993). While much of this activity related to market forces, it drew as well from financial incentives under Medicare's Prospective Payment System (PPS) and the indemnity plans, which adopted similar measures. By placing a prospective budget on funds for particular care episodes in hospitals, PPS encouraged hospitals to do more procedures on an outpatient basis and to discharge patients earlier. Having other providers at hand to pick up this "before" and "after" care meant the potential for greater total corporate revenues and flexibility.

This type of care management also required greater financial accountability and service coordination for individual cases. Not surprisingly, case management began to appear in new care settings, particularly institutional ones; it also became part of managerial strategies collectively termed *managed care* as well as private sector initiatives. The next sections review these developments as they have affected care for older people.

Back to the Institution

Case management has become part of the acute care hospital through several applications. New technologies referred to as *critical paths, clinical pathways,* or *care mapping* outline core care requirements as well as associated staff actions and key interventions for patients with particular diagnoses, based on a target time line. In and of themselves, these techniques represent a form of care coordination, which is often placed under the supervision of a case manager. In tertiary care hospitals, case management guides care delivery of multidisciplinary service or product lines, such as women's health, surgery, or rehabilitative services; here, all inpatients are assigned care teams with a case manager, and critical paths direct care delivery. Primary nurses generally occupy these types of case management positions (Satinsky, 1995).

More directly related to care of the elderly are hospital-based geriatric case management programs for managing high-risk, high-cost Medicare patients and case management systems for monitoring elderly patients' outcomes following discharge, which are attempts to integrate acute and long-term care services in a care package (Read & O'Brien, 1989; Satinsky, 1995; Wimberley & Blazyk, 1989). One early leader in this regard was the Robert Wood Johnson Foundation Program for Hospital Initiatives in Long-Term Care, which ran 24 demonstration projects providing interdisciplinary team case management to recently discharged elderly patients and those at risk of hospital or nursing home admission (Coombs, Eisdorfer, Feiden, & Kessler, 1989; MacAdam et al., 1989). Case management has also become part of efforts to develop comprehensive geriatric care programs within skilled nursing homes, again in response to the changes toward admitting sicker patients for shorter-term stays (Burton, 1994; Lowery, 1995).

At first glance, locating case management within a health care institution, making that setting central to service delivery, appears contradictory to the founding goals of community-based care case management—most particularly the goal of preventing institutionalization. Yet, in both types of programs, case management is primarily concerned with achieving the most appropriate and comprehensive care plan, including institutional care when essential and effective. And both types can ill afford to ignore the cost-effectiveness of such plans, whether or not they operate under a capitated or risk-bearing structure. There may, in short, be little difference today in the care plans devised by programs centered in institutional settings and those of programs in the community—other than where the case contact begins.

On the other hand, there remain subtle but important differences between the priorities of institutional comprehensive case-managed care programs and those that remain focused on increasing access to community-based services. The orientation of hospital case management toward institutional goals is well captured in a book recently published by an affiliate of the American Hospital Association:

> As health care organizations and services are combined and reshaped, and as methods of payment encourage less instead of more use of the health care system, health care professionals have an opportunity to ease the transition by means of applying a case management approach to service delivery. . . . Case managers . . . can be valuable resources who are aware of, and have access to, a variety of options for care. They can encourage the use of tools such as clinical paths to help appropriate clinicians deliver care efficiently. They can use outcome data to assess the effectiveness of the delivery process. Because they do not have the responsibility for providing direct care, they can spend time developing relationships and networks. Armed with a vast knowledge of resources, they also can be effective patient advocates. (Satinsky, 1995, pp. 1, 3)

If not entirely an afterthought, patient advocacy and service brokerage clearly take second place here to goals of cost containment and quality assessment. These goals find further expression in the uses of case management within managed care.

Case Management and Managed Care

As concerns about health care costs intensified through the latter half of the 1980s, both public and private sectors embraced managed care strategies for cost containment. Practically synonymous with health maintenance organizations (HMOs) until this point, the term *managed care* henceforth would denote a variety of programs and structures aimed at improving service efficiency, coordinating service delivery, and controlling utilization, particularly by reducing use of services deemed inappropriate or excessive. Many of these programs relied on case managers to serve as the key functionaries working toward those ends.

Under managed care, case management incorporates institutional as well as community-based service settings; its practitioners include more physicians or nurse specialists who may or may not have direct contact with patients. Case management here often narrows to a form of rationing of more extensive and expensive forms of care, though it can also be part of attempts to provide comprehensive care packages.

Though federal policy had supported HMO development for years before, a more direct public foray into managed care came with changes in federal law in the Omnibus Budget Reconciliation Act (OBRA) of 1981. It was, of course, OBRA that first facilitated the community-based care initiatives discussed previously. Among the other alternative financing and delivery approaches OBRA permitted were several enabling contracts with HMOs for Medicaid services and the authorization for states to establish Primary Care Case Management (PCCM) systems for Medicaid recipients. While many aspects of case management varied among states, common to all the PCCM programs is the requirement that Medicaid recipients go to their case managers (who are either physicians or primary care clinics) for all direct primary care and through the case manager authorization process for other services (Freund & Neuschler, 1986; Hurley & Fennell, 1990).

Though most PCCM programs did not cover long-term care or the institutionalized elderly, by 1990, Medicaid programs in nine states more directly targeted elders living in the community for inclusion in managed care programs through contracts with HMOs. While the consolidation of services in HMOs was itself a form of case management, some states used additional case management services to coordinate long-term care services with the more acute care reimbursed under Medicare. Managed care also reached older Americans through HMOs contracting to Medicare. By 1991, HMO risk contracts were the principal form of managed care under Medicare, though they still enrolled a small proportion of Medicare recipients (Spitz & Abramson, 1987).

In addition to separate initiatives under Medicaid and Medicare, the push to develop coordinated care programs led HCFA to sponsor two sets of demonstration programs consolidating acute and long-term care services within managed care environments: On Lok and the PACE demonstrations, and the Social Health Maintenance Organization (S/HMO) programs.

From its beginnings in the early 1970s as a demonstration day health center in San Francisco's North Beach/Chinatown district, On Lok steadily expanded its service capacity and funding streams, developing innovations looked to as models for long-term care systems (see N. A. Miller, 1992; Zawadski & Eng, 1988). Over time, the program began to target very frail elders, making available to them a full contingent of social and medical services in home, community-based, and institutional settings, with case management provided by interdisciplinary teams. In 1983, the program assumed financial risk for client care by shifting from cost-based reimbursement to capitation based on fixed monthly premiums, in the process including Medicare, Medicaid, and private pay among its funding sources.

The program's ability to assume risk while augmenting the service system for a vulnerable population sufficiently impressed federal policymakers that the Omnibus Reconciliation Act of 1986 authorized replication of the On Lok model at 10 sites; further legislation in 1990 increased this to 15 sites, termed the Program of All-inclusive Care for the Elderly (PACE). Nine sites continued to operate through the mid-1990s under capitated payment systems. All targeted nursing-home-eligible clients, provided a range of community-based long-term care services through adult day health centers, operated through capitated Medicare and Medicaid reimbursements, and used multidisciplinary teams for case management (Branch, Coulam, & Zimmerman, 1995).

The second consolidated service approach was that of Social Health Maintenance Organizations (S/HMOs), which ran as HCFA demonstrations from 1985 to 1992, with some continuing under different organizational auspices. S/HMOs were prepaid, vertically integrated systems of care incorporating the "full range of ambulatory, acute inpatient, rehabilitative, nursing home, home health, and personal care services under a prospectively determined fixed budget" (Greenberg, Leutz, & Altman, 1989, p. 197). Some were situated in HMOs, others in long-term care organizations. Case management in the S/HMO had a broader role and scope of authority than in earlier community-based care demonstrations since case managers assumed the main responsibility, as well as fiscal accountability, in authorizing and monitoring long-term care services (Yordi, 1988).

A final way in which case management has become a core managed care technology affecting the elderly is as a cost containment strategy in indemnity insurance plans for high-cost cases, which often involve persons affected by multiple organ failures or chronic care needs. By the early 1990s about two-thirds of the large private indemnity plans used case management for this purpose; most health care benefits management firms and many small independent plans have also adopted this approach (Wallack, 1991). Case managers are generally registered nurses (sometimes with specialized training in specific diagnostic or rehabilitation areas), who focus on chart reviews and have minimal, if any, patient contact (Henderson, Souder, Bergman, & Collard, 1988); the major objective of case management here is to achieve the delivery of a "lower intensity" of care (Wallack, 1991, p. 29), clearly a more limited role than the comprehensive forms of case management reviewed previously.

Going Private: Professional and Consumer Approaches

While case management expanded in medical and managed care settings as part of efforts to increase market competitiveness, it has also become a market commodity itself. Two distinct signs of this are the rise of private practice case management and the move toward client-centered or consumer-directed programs.

In the late 1970s and early 1980s, many professional-level case managers, who had been drawn in the first place to the more clinical aspects of case management, initiated practices offering private case management on a fee-for-service basis (Austin, 1990). Private services were thus highly professionalized; a national survey of private case management providers in the late 1980s found that over one-third employed only Masters-level social works (MSWs), with close to two-thirds employing at least one MSW case manager. The offerings of these services—commonly including financial assessment, psychotherapy, financial counseling, and estate management—clearly aimed at a private-pay market (Secord, 1987, reported in Austin, 1990).

The strength of private practice case management for the elderly is evident in the founding of the National Association of Professional Geriatric Care Managers (NAPGCM) in the mid-1980s. The association has become an active promoter of the trade, publishing a *Geriatric Care Management Journal* and issuing case management standards as early as 1990 (NAPGCM, 1992). In alliance with an academic research center named the Case Management Institute, NAPGCM also established a National Academy of Certified Care Managers, a seven-member board of experts charged with developing a credentialing process for care managers in long-term care, chronic care, and the disabilities field (Quinn, 1994; Geron & Chassler, 1994).

While these trends, with others reviewed later, suggest the increased professionalism of case management, a countertrend has been the growing emphasis on having clients manage their own care. These client-centered, or consumer-driven approaches draw from many policy currents. One source is the legacy of the structural changes that followed Medicare's Prospective Payment System: Hospitals discharged patients in sicker conditions and with more care needs to both nursing home and home settings, and home care became even more a form of medical care than it had been under the already medically oriented Medicare coverage (Estes et al., 1993). The home became the site for therapeutic interventions once confined to institutional walls, including chemotherapy, intravenous drug treatment, and renal dialysis. This "medicalization" of the home placed increased personal care burdens on patients and their family members, while Medicare coverage remained largely limited to more skilled forms of therapy.

There was a growing gap between the model of home care sanctioned by public funding and the functional care needs of elders at home. This was even more the case for working-age adults with disabilities. In the late 1970s, the independent living movement arose among groups of disabled adults seeking to make their physical as well as social environments better suited to their needs, instead of forcing their adaptation to nonsupportive environments. A large focus of this movement was on a new model of home care, a model centered on personal care services provided by attendants selected, trained, and supervised by the care recipient. Eschewing such terms as *attendant, client,* and even *care* as embodying a normalization of dependency and professional control, the proponents of this model called for consumer-directed "personal assistance" services (Batavia, De-Jong, & McKnew, 1991).

This model clearly differed from that of home care in the domain of long-term care for the elderly, a difference not merely of words but of both the philosophy and the structure of care (Simon-Rusinowitz & Hofland, 1993; see also the comparison with peer-modeling strategies in Albrecht & Peters, 1997). Since the mid-1980s, disability advocates have met with leaders in the aging field to try to reconcile those differences and develop a common agenda. While it is still the former leading the push for a national personal assistance program (as proposed, for example, by the National Council on the Handicapped in 1986 and by the World Institute on Disability in 1989 [Simon-Rusinowitz & Hofland, 1993]), there are increasing calls within elder care for more consumer-directed approaches.

One such initiative is a four-state demonstration project sponsored by the Robert Wood Johnson Foundation (Mahoney & Simon-Rusinowitz, 1997). The Cash and Counseling Demonstration and Evaluation gives consumers (both elders and working-age adults with disabilities) the option of cash payments to purchase their own personal assistance services, with counseling to help clients make informed decisions about program options. Case management here clearly rests with the consumer, a move in line with the interests of state officials, who, concerned with "achieving program economies," have begun to notice that "case management can be expensive" and to question "whether it should be universally required" (Ibid, p. 26). At the same time, there is room for case management organizations here to provide the counseling of consumers, as well as to share in the responsibility of care management. A similar mixture is part of the new Independent Living Training Program offered through the Paralyzed Veterans of America, which offers an option of professional case management in a program of services determined by the consumer (Gilson & Casebolt, 1997). To the extent that these approaches incorporate formal case management, they thus require of it an advocacy role focused on client empowerment.

It is clear that this movement represents a thrust apart from the mainstream in long-term care case management, which, though paying more attention to client preferences, remains firmly under professional direction. Indicative of this are recent signs of increased professionalism in the field fostered by associations such as the National Association of Professional

Geriatric Care Managers (NAPGCM), which is one of several groups that have developed professional standards and/or certification criteria for long-term care case management. Others include the National Council on Aging, the National Association of Social Workers, and the National Advisory Committee on Long-Term Care Case Management, sponsored by the Robert Wood Johnson Foundation (Geron & Chassler, 1994). Efforts in the early 1990s to legislate a national long-term care insurance program explain part of the momentum to define case management as a professional enterprise (United States General Accounting Office [USGAO], 1993).

Beyond standards and certification, the professionalization of long-term care case management is evident in an array of dedicated journals and conferences. Joan Quinn (whose career, as director first of Triage, then of Connecticut Community Care, Inc., and now of managed care initiatives for a major health care insurer, parallels case management's own evolution) founded the *Journal of Case Management* in 1991. NAPGCM publishes its own trade journal on the topic. The American Society on Aging, whose members largely come from long-term care practice, has sponsored a yearly International Conference on Long-Term Care Case Management since 1993, and a variety of related institutional conferences take place annually.

These efforts to establish practice standards and professional discourse certainly enhance the legitimacy of case management as a service technology, but we still know very little about how (or how well) that technology works in practice. That is, we still have not looked very far into the workings of the black box. A recent report by the National Advisory Committee on Long-Term Care Case Management reveals how little we still know about basic aspects of case management practice when it identifies the following questions as "warranting immediate research or consideration":

- How do costs and consumer outcomes vary with the intensity, duration, and scope of case management activities?
- Who needs what level of case management?
- Who should do case management? What are the skills and competencies needed to perform case management?
- How does case management practice currently vary across settings and practice applications?
- What staffing levels and methods of contact are most effective?
- What are the likely effects of anticipated technological changes and alternative service delivery systems such as managed care on case management practice? (Geron & Chassler, 1995, p. 13)

That almost 30 years of case management program expansion and diffusion could occur without answers to these questions is, indeed, remarkable. The next section explores how this could have happened.

Suspending Disbelief: Explaining Case
Management's Enduring Popularity

There are at least two simple reasons why case management spread and prospered in the long-term sector despite the lack of consistent evidence of its efficiency and effectiveness. First, questions of the type raised by the National Advisory Committee were never the ones of greatest concern— to policymakers, program officers, or evaluation researchers. Only in the Channeling experiment and a few crosscutting program evaluations was there a systematic attempt to examine the significance of different forms of case management practice. As a line of research, moreover, evaluating what case managers did and how they did it required an intense, even messy form of data collection over and above more easily measured outcome variables.

In this regard, consider a summary assessment of the lessons of long-term care demonstrations and Medicaid waiver programs offered by Robert Applebaum, a gerontologist long involved in the community care movement:

> We have learned that chronically disabled people with severe disability can receive services in their own homes with no negative effects on physical functioning, health, and longevity. We have learned that even when in-home services have been expanded considerably, families remain key providers of care. . . . We have learned that, when provided with a choice, the vast majority of consumers prefer to receive services at home rather than in an institutional setting, and this increases consumer quality of life. We have learned the level of services that people need to function adequately in the community, and how much these services and the accompanying case management service cost to deliver. Finally, we have learned that long-term care is much more varied than we had expected, with considerable fluctuation in the condition of the consumer, the type and amount of services needed, and the length of time case-managed in-home care is needed. (Applebaum, 1996, p. 90)

A second relatively simple reason is that case management was riding the policy tides of the times. Cast as a neutral service technology, it easily accommodated the objectives of service access and availability of the late 1960s and early '70s, of cost containment and resource allocation from the mid-'70s to mid-'80s, and of service consolidation and fiscal accountability from the mid-'80s to the present. If it, or the programs using it, could not be proven to be the best way to advance particular objectives, neither did it greatly undermine them. Case managed community-based care, for instance, could be claimed at least to be no more (or not exceptionally more) expensive than nursing home care, while providing a service generally preferred by clients and families to entering a nursing home[15]. (Applebaum, 1996)

Simple explanations are incomplete, however, because they fail to acknowledge the role played by those actively promoting case management in the context of an evolving sequence of service programs. At the level of the service community, from the early 1970s on, this included all the nonprofit health and social service agencies providing diverse forms of community-based care programs as well as state and local governmental offices involved in their funding. The growth of the home care industry alone over the next 20 years—from 208 provider agencies in 1961 to over 6,000 certified home health agencies and 8,000 noncertified providers by 1987 (Applebaum & Flint, 1993)—suggests how easily case management could spread from demonstration status to a standard program feature. Each new community-based program invested not only in the practice of case management, but also in doing it in the way thought most responsive to the demands and contingencies of its local environment.

In turn, this variability reinforced broader policy favoring local and state autonomy in program design, a trend in evidence early on in case management's history and no less evident today. This emphasis is most recently apparent in the conclusion of a 1993 General Accounting Office (GAO) report on case management standards that

> Because of variations in state and local organizational structures, economic situations, geography, and client demographics, we believe that, if the Congress desires to have federal standards, broad standards similar to those already established by organizations like NCOA or NASW would be most appropriate. We believe that specific details concerning how the case management process is to operate and the qualifications case managers should possess are best determined at the state and local level. (USGAO, 1993, pp. 39–40)

Despite the rhetoric of advocacy, particularly in early programs, case management does not challenge the service status quo nor demand major structural change. The GAO formulation uses the variability of case management itself as evidence supporting the maintenance of nonstandardized systems of care.

As case management spread beyond the community care movement, this variability would increase, and its constituents similarly diffused, particularly within the field of medical care. Ties to managed care, institutional care planning, private practice, and the independent living movement meant that new proponents would be advancing the use of case management on new playing fields.

It is essential to understand case management's status as a service technology as a symbolic resource for these players, not merely a form of practice they help to develop. By claiming a need for better assessment and "targeting," proponents of community care could keep alive the push for more case-managed demonstrations even when initial ones were less than successful. The call for immediate research quoted previously can be seen in the same light, as can attempts to develop case management guidelines. What each of these does is to propose that there are technological solutions for the current failings of case management programs. Challenges from the independent living movement suggest, in contrast, that what may be amiss is not the solution, but rather that we are asking the wrong question—namely, how to fix a service system built on fundamentally flawed assumptions and structures. At the same time, consumer-centered care has become the latest technological twist in case management circles (and health care, in general), with providers seeing client responsibility as one way to reconcile concerns about autonomy and choice with means of controlling costs (Scala, Mayberry, & Kunkel, 1996).

Two sources of case management's continued legitimacy, then, have been the efforts of its expanding groups of supporters and their success in linking case management to key policy objectives through claims about its status as a service technology. Supporters have invoked, as well, claims of professional status. This, too, plays into issues of local autonomy, since, in advancing local discretion, providers can also assert professional decision making. The professional claims for case managers have become more pronounced in response to the threats to the professional nature of case management work that come with increased use of caremaps and clinical decision-making algorithms. Quests for an accepted knowledge base, standards of training and practice, and certification credentials are, as one long-term observer and proponent of case management put it, "normal evolutionary steps" in this process of professionalization (Applebaum, 1996, p. 90).

Even if its proponents ground the legitimacy of a program in technological and professional claims, in practice that program must recreate its own legitimation on a daily basis—that is, it must maintain its legitimacy in the eyes of its staff, clients, and other constituents. Looking over the history of case management programs, despite all their structural permutations, two relatively constant attributes suggest ways in which programs sustain this legitimacy. The first is that core staff mainly consist of service professionals, especially nurses and social workers, sometimes teamed with physicians and / or paraprofessional assistants. Allied with this, the fundamental form of long-term care case management is provider-driven in that the case managers construct, direct, supervise, and administer the plan of care (Batavia et al., 1991). Professional forms of knowledge and practice are thus likely to be critically related to the way case managers construct the case, and in turn to their legitimation of program operations.

The second fixture of case management programs serving the elderly is that their fundamental function is one of linking clients to services. For the most part, case managers themselves do not provide these services directly; what varies among programs is the extent of their ability to authorize services provided by others. Attempts to see what difference such resource control makes, as in the Channeling demonstration, have provided tantalizing suggestions that case management functions, including the definition of client need, change as this structure changes; but there is little research evidence to expand on those suggestions. It is at least worth speculating, however, that the way case management programs sustain legitimacy has to do with their relationships with other service providers and what those relationships mean for clients.

The final section examines the implications of these aspects of practice by looking at the actual operations of a case management program.

CASE MANAGEMENT IN PRACTICE

During one winter of the [case management] Project's operation, Mr. Valducci was being pressured to pay an overdue heating bill. The bill was high, in part, because heating the house was complicated by a hole in the roof. The Project had gotten an agreement from his union to cover the cost of repairing the roof, but Mr. Valducci rejected the money, saying the union should increase his pension instead. The Project's next strategy was to get Mr. Valducci an application for public assistance with the heating bills. Though unable to write, he balked at having the case managers complete the form for him, saying he'd "let them know" if he wanted their help. . . . He said his main reason for remaining in his house was his son, who for years had been in a mental institution. Though he acknowledged that he never expected his son to come out, he stated, "but this is still his home." . . . The nurse [case manager] stated at one point regarding the hole in Mr. Valducci's roof, "At least it's in his dining room. He doesn't go in there much." (Adapted from Dill, 1990, pp. 241–242)

What is case management in practice? This is a deceptively simple question, and as noted previously, one seldom addressed in evaluations of case management programs. It is relatively easy to think of ways to describe what case managers do; for example, the size of their caseloads, the breadth of the services they provide, and the duration of their involvement with clients are all good indicators of the comprehensiveness of their services (see Applebaum & Austin, 1990). It is also simple to identify and measure some outcomes of case managers' actions, such as the completion of reassessments or service referrals. None of these measures tells us much about *how* case managers do their work, however, or about the dilemmas they face in their relationships with clients.

Studies that examine case management practice generally rely on self-reports by case managers about how often they perform particular activities or how they allocate their work time (e.g., White & Grisham, 1982; Schneider, Hirsch, Galper, Rickards, & Sterthous, 1984; cf. Kane & Kane, 1987). There has also been analysis of the ethical and practice dilemmas case managers commonly face (Kane & Caplan, 1993; Clemens, Wetle, Feltes, Crabtree, & Dubitzky, 1994). These approaches get us closer to understanding what it is case managers actually do, but still fail to capture the dynamics of how they do it. Similarly, recent efforts to identify best-practice techniques in long-term care case management (e.g., Geron & Chassler, 1994, 1995) cull optimal practices from decades of program experience but leave undocumented the actual practices and experiences of the case managers.

One reason for the lack of attention to this area is that the contingencies that complicate case management practice also confound attempts to describe it. How can objective, reliable research describe a process driven by the idiosyncratic needs of clients and bounded by the specific nature of particular service systems? And what would be the generalizability of such a description? To answer both questions, we need to see case management in a broader conceptual framework; that is, as one example of a category of services and organizations which perform similar functions in similar ways.

In seeking to give their clients access to services, and thus make them clients of other providers as well, case management programs conform to what sociologist Yeheskel Hasenfeld (1972) terms a "people-processing organization." Unlike organizations such as hospitals, jails, and schools, which try to change people's lives or behavior directly, people-processing organizations have as a primary goal to process people into a new public status. Examples include diagnostic clinics, employment placement services, and university admissions offices. The sequence of tasks through which they do this processing bears a striking resemblance to the stages of case management: assessment of the client, exploration of alternate services or placements, choice of appropriate action, and managing the clients' relocation (Hasenfeld, 1972). Many of the line positions in this type of organization involve boundary-spanning and brokerage activities concerned with controlling people's access to different social settings and with mediating relations between clients and other organizations.

Seeing case management as a boundary-spanning role in a people-processing organization gives us a framework to compare how case management practice works in different service settings. To illustrate this, I will

draw from research I conducted on two case management programs serving elderly persons (Dill, 1986).

A Tale of Two Programs

The programs described in the following were two parts of a community
care project that operated from 1980 to 1984 at a social service agency in a
major Northeast metropolitan area. The "Project" had a caseload of 250
clients who were over 60 and judged to be homebound. The Project's overall objective was to coordinate home care and other services needed to
maintain clients in the community. The two component parts used different means toward that end. One, which I term *CM*, performed mainly referral and advocacy activities, acting as a broker of services for clients. The
other, *CM+*, provided clients with homemaker services, transportation to
medical care, and payment for prescription drugs under Medicare waivers.
Case managers in both CM and CM+ consisted of teams of a nurse and a
social worker (though CM+ also used paraprofessional workers to coordinate service arrangements and billing), and their formal job descriptions
were essentially the same, encompassing assessment, care planning, service implementation, and monitoring functions.[16]

Understanding the Project as a people-processing organization helps us
see, first of all, that an important force shaping case management practice
consists of relations with the other agencies to which clients were being
"processed," that is, the ones from which services were being sought. For
CM+, the focal point of case management was on the provision of
waivered services, namely, homemakers, transportation, and pharmaceu-
ticals. The case management staff did not routinely develop linkages with
organizations beyond those contracted with for those services. More particularly, the emphasis in case management was on the homemaker service
because of the many contingencies involved in assigning homemakers and
mediating their relationships with clients.

The assignment of homemakers was negotiated on a daily basis between the project and the agency employing the homemakers. Factors in-
fluencing those assignments added a layer of informal criteria to those
formally used in developing a care plan to meet clients' needs. The geographic location of clients, for example, frequently determined which
homemaker would be assigned and for what hours. Clients in areas not
well served by public transportation might have to wait several weeks for
a homemaker, and then get one on days when that person happened to be
assigned to another client in the same area.

The case managers also focused on mediating the relationship between
clients and homemakers ("managing the client's relocation," in theoretical
terms). This became apparent in case conferences held with the case man-

agers by the project director, as from one-half to two-thirds of the cases discussed in a particular meeting involved issues related to homemakers. These ranged from simple problems with homemakers' schedules to complex problems in the homemakers' relationships with clients and their families. Such problems often led to case managers explaining to each side the appropriate role expectations of the other. The case of "Mrs. Bonati" (as drawn from notes from a case conference) illustrates how case managers defined the homemaker role through negotiation with the client's informal caregiver:

> Mrs. Bonati, a client in her late 80s, lives on the first floor of a house owned by a relative whom she refers to as a "niece." While she has several chronic conditions, she is considered to be functioning well and not "at risk" of institutionalization. The homemaker reports being finished with the work requested of her after three hours of her four-hour shift. She complains that the "niece" will not let her watch television with the client and has removed an extension phone from the apartment to keep the homemaker from using it. The staff feel the homemaker is important as a companion to Mrs. Bonati. The social worker will try to persuade the niece to replace the telephone and allow the homemaker to watch television when her work is finished. She will also discuss with the niece the nature of the "companion" role.

Case managers could also be called upon to interpret the "client" role to homemakers, as in the case of "Mrs. Cumberland":

> Mrs. Cumberland, a client in her 80s, had a stroke two years ago. Until then, she had been very active and lived on her own; now she lives with her daughter. Although she has been receiving speech therapy and physiotherapy, she has not made any progress in her recovery within the past year. The homemaker had called the staff because Mrs. Cumberland had been angry and crying and had told the homemaker to call her daughter home from work and then leave. This was the third homemaker assigned to Mrs. Cumberland, the two previous ones having left under conditions of mutual dissatisfaction. The nurse views Mrs. Cumberland's outbursts (of which this is but the latest) as reflecting emotional lability subsequent to her stroke and plateau in recovery. She will talk to the homemaker to explain Mrs. Cumberland's physical condition and discuss ways to manage her.

These examples help us understand that the way case management practice defines a *case* only partially consists of attributes of the individual client. Casework in CM+ centered, additionally, on the relationships among clients, their informal caregivers, and formal service providers. Indeed, ensuring the smooth operation of those dyadic or triadic units defined the essence of the management of the case.

Where CM+ represents the service authorization model of case management, CM illustrates the brokerage model in which case managers neither provide nor control service resources. Since they depended entirely on other programs to provide care for their clients, it is not surprising that these case managers focused their efforts on identifying alternate service possibilities, deciding among them, and attempting to implement them. Once services were in place, their job was largely done, since they had little ability to intervene between the client and the other service provider.

Case managers in CM maintained much wider contacts within their service community than did those in CM+. They listed over 20 agencies, of a variety of types, with which they tried to maintain working relations. The main purpose of these relations was to provide an ongoing source of information about service eligibility and availability; while such information gathering was unrelated to the needs of particular cases, case managers could use what they learned for any case should the need arise. The salience of this knowledge base is indicated by the fact that in staff conferences observed over a 7-month period, case managers raised issues related to the services provided by particular agencies in over 70% of the cases they discussed.

The network of agencies to which CM made referrals was equally broad. The largest proportion of referrals was for homemaker services, for which clients generally had to pay privately. Since such payment was beyond the means of many clients, CM staff also "unbundled" the services a homemaker could provide, attempting to meet the same needs through a variety of programs. A volunteer program, for example, could help with shopping errands, housecleaning, and laundry; meals-on-wheels could deliver meals; direct deposit and mail services could accomplish banking activities; companionship and recreation could be found in adult education programs and senior centers.

One of the main tasks the CM case managers had was to cultivate good working relationships with staff at those other agencies. An example of how this could help with client processing concerns Medicaid entitlements. Though the criteria for determining Medicaid eligibility appeared standardized and inflexible, case managers found there was latitude given Medicaid staff in interpreting those criteria. Thus, some Medicaid workers were more likely than others to accept the case managers' presentation of the client, without asking for exhaustive independent documentation, or to give the case manager the benefit of a doubt in evaluating a case. Case managers tried to develop ongoing relations with such workers, bypassing the "first available worker" basis for assignment when they entered the Medicaid office. The benefits of this were illustrated by the delight expressed by one of the case managers in being able to get approval of Medicaid for a client in the remarkably short span of two weeks. The Medicaid worker, one she had dealt with on previous cases, told her she would "forget about" a bank book showing the client had savings in excess of that allowed; she suggested that the client set up a separate burial account with these funds, which would be an allowable resource. Once she saw that this had been done, she approved and processed the application.

Because CM lacked the ability to authorize or control homemaker services, its case managers did not become involved in mediating the homemaker / client relationship the way those in CM+ did. Indeed, issues related to homemaker activities or the client / homemaker relationship arose in only 7% of the cases discussed in case conferences. This lack of involvement also meant that CM's staff had little ability to influence the behavior of staff at the agencies that did provide homemakers to their clients. A specific instance in which this frustrated the staff was in their efforts to obtain weekly progress notes filed by homemakers in the agency which received the most referrals (which still numbered less than 25) from the Project. Although the agency verbally agreed to supply those reports, it never systematically forwarded them. CM+, in contrast, was a central collection point for homemakers' reports on clients.

On a positive note, by unbundling the homemaker role, CM was able to target care specifically to clients' needs. On the other hand, having to secure different services and diverse sources of payment for them led to a patchwork form of case management, with much staff activity directed toward seeking and coordinating care. These activities were complicated by the multiple and interactive nature of the very needs that prompted them, such that one situation could not be addressed without addressing others, as the case of "Mrs. Tower" suggests:

> Mrs. Tower, a client in her 70s, is terminally ill with cancer; she also has heart and pulmonary disease. Currently living with her daughter, she realizes her condition is deteriorating and wishes to enter a nursing home. Neither she nor her daughter has the resources to pay for this privately. Although Mrs. Tower parted from her husband some time ago, she never obtained a legal separation. Until she is legally separated, her ability to claim Medicaid coverage will be circumscribed by her husband's financial status. Her husband is unwilling to provide money for her care, but is also unwilling to cooperate with separation proceedings. Mrs. Tower's daughter contacted the Legal Aid office for help in obtaining a legal separation, and her case has been on their waiting list. The CM social worker will contact a Legal Aid lawyer specializing in cases involving older people in an attempt to expedite the case. In the meantime, the staff are trying to find home care services, and payment for them, since the daughter has obtained a part-time job and Mrs. Tower will be left alone a few hours each day. They have arranged for the local branch of the Cancer Society to provide a homemaker on a time-limited basis. The social worker is also checking on the possibility of receiving coverage of home care from a union to which Mrs. Tower's husband belongs.

As this case shows, case management in CM involved taking apart the statuses and identities of clients, then reconstructing and packaging them in a way that would secure services. This meant that the definition of the *case* was more variable and dynamic than in CM+: At any given time, the focus of casework could be on only a small segment of a client's life, on all of it, or on a unit that included other actors as well. Moreover, that focus shifted among these modes over time in response to what was available in the service environment as well as changes in the client's need.

So far we have seen that what case management is in practice depends not only on the attributes of clients but also on the structure of the case management program and its relationships with other provider agencies. Whether a particular agency will matter enough to a case management program to develop an ongoing working relationship will, of course, depend on the nature of the goals, services, eligibility criteria, and target population of each. In addition, the impact of an outside agency on case management will depend on the structure of the relationship: the extent to which each depends on the other for clients or services, the extent to which alternative sources are available, and the degree of restrictiveness or discretion each can exert in choosing among those alternatives thus become critical factors in defining case management in practice.

To understand this process, consider again the tasks involved in the way people-processing organizations evaluate and process clients: client assessment, exploration of alternate services, choice of appropriate action, and management of clients' relocation. The structure and quality of a case management program's relationship with other agencies can shape any one of these tasks in practice (cf. Albrecht & Peters, 1995). When a case management program can authorize a service resource, as was the case with CM+, contractual arrangements preclude the need to examine alternative services and reach a decision in each case. The main tasks for case management practice thus become evaluating the fit of the client with the services to be provided and mediating the relationship once those services begin. With a brokerage model such as CM, in which case managers neither provide nor control direct services, the eligibility requirements of an important agency might be added to client assessment instruments or informally shape the attention case managers give to the placement of clients there. The needs of clients and the characteristics of the case management program are thus not as separable as the use of objective needs assessment instruments makes them seem.

Advocates of a purely brokerage model of case management argued that it would subject case managers least to a conflict of interest between their roles as client advocates and as employees of a service provider organization concerned with the costs and effectiveness of care. But we have seen here that the way case managers define and manage the *case* is inherently shaped by what they can do or provide for the client, which in turn is framed by the structure of their organization and its relations with others. In this regard, there is likely to be little difference between brokerage and service authorization models of case management. Even in models in which the case management program directly provides care or has more fiscal control, we would expect to find feedback between the nature of case managers' linkages with the direct service providers and the ways they define and respond to the needs of clients. Constrained service resources and pressures for cost containment in particular introduce conflict with the commonly voiced philosophy of client-centered case management (Clemens et al., 1994).

The question then is not how to isolate case management from organizational interests (whether those of their own or another agency), since that cannot be done, given the basic structure of the case manager role. Rather, the challenge is how to ensure that organizational interests do not override those of serving clients in a manner they themselves prefer. One way in which case managers address this dilemma is by using their professional expertise to provide care responding first and foremost to clients' needs and preferences. Case managers attempt to define and understand clients' needs and preferences in terms of models based in their professions, in the process designating their work as a professional undertaking. Since the goals of case management programs center on meeting these professionally defined needs, the use of professional models creates the semblance of unity between client interests and organizational interests. Defining what is in clients' best interests in terms of these professional understandings may, however, conflict with other views of those interests, including those of the clients themselves. The next section examines this and other practice implications of case management as a professional role.

The Professional Gaze

We have seen how case management in long-term care has been performed mainly by social workers and nurses. Case management in practice reflects the substance and standards of those disciplines, even when case managers do not directly provide social work or nursing care for their clients. Assessment instruments, for example, typically include indicators of the client's social, mental, and physical well-being—measures of social activity, social support, physical and mental functioning, health care needs, and so forth. Even more, the practice of case management incorporates the bodies of knowledge, models, ideologies, and tacit assumptions comprising those professions, building them into the fabric of the work case managers do.

In looking at case management in the CM+ project, I described how case managers interpreted the role of homemaker to clients and in turn mediated homemakers' interpretations of clients. Going back to those cases, we can see that the case managers were drawing on professional models in negotiating the client-homemaker relationship: the psychosocial model of companion with Mrs. Bonati and the biomedical model of stroke recovery with Mrs. Cumberland. This indicates that the control case managers have in defining the role of homemaker or client goes beyond their ability to authorize and pay for the service. It lies as well in their ability to use their professional expertise in controlling how the reality of the case is to be understood by both parties. In turn, mediating in this way between clients and homemakers reproduces and reinforces that expertise as an essential component of case management practice.

Although professional models provide a latent or "available" culture that case managers can draw on at any point, they most clearly shape needs assessment and care-planning activities. In Chapter 1, we saw how the model of *need* used in human service systems reflects professional ideologies and interests developed since the Progressive Era. Elsewhere (Dill, 1993) I have shown how formal assessment procedures in case management identify need in terms of what individual clients lack (as classified in professionally defined categories) that can be remedied through professional action. In this approach, the needy individual is a care recipient rather than an agent in the production of the process by which care is delivered. Clients' own understandings of their lives and needs enter this process only to the extent they fit within the framework of the needs assessment; perspectives that do not fit in those frames are systematically marginalized or excluded as noise in the proper functioning of the assessment process.

In addition to formal assessment procedures, case managers develop what I term informal, clinical perspectives on cases, using their clinical training and experience to evaluate the pathological implications of various aspects of client's lives (Dill, 1990). The perspectives of the nurse and social worker case managers I studied varied in predictable ways, with nurses more focused on physical functioning and medical conditions and social workers, on social relationships and social psychological issues. In case conferences, the contrast between these perspectives could be startling:

Project Coordinator (PC): What about Mrs. D.?
Nurse (N): She has had Parkinson's and can't even hold on to the stair rail. Her daughter's still living there [because the client needs so much help].
Social Worker (SW): Her main problem is that she has to show her children that she's failing. She hates to be a burden to them.
PC: Mrs. M.?

N: She's getting eight hours a week of [homemaker] service. She has a pace-maker and a colostomy.

SW: She's resourceful, has lots of interests. She enjoys her home and knits and reads.

PC: The Cs [a couple]?

SW: They're terrific, wonderful, very supportive of each other.

N: He has poor mental status [due to] CVAs [strokes]. He's incontinent, needs lot of care. Mrs. C. won't take more than eight hours [of homemaker service]. . . . She says, 'I have to keep busy.'

On the one hand, the fact that different professional orientations yield variable reports of clients' situations argues strongly for the type of inter-disciplinary team approach commonly found in long-term care case man-agement. On the other hand, combining the clinical viewpoint of a nurse with that of a social worker clearly does not produce an *inter*disciplinary perspective. It does, however, make more professional "cultures" avail-able for use in defining clients' needs and deciding what services are ap-propriate.

One of the persistent findings in medical sociology and medical an-thropology has been that such professional cultures only partially overlap with the systems of meanings, values, and norms of laypeople (Freidson, 1970; Conrad, 1985; Kleinman, 1978). Critics charge that when care pro-grams adopt a professional stance, they place service recipients in an in-herently dependent position, compromising their rights to care and their ability to control service delivery (Lloyd, 1991; Estes, 1993). Part of this de-pendency derives from the fact that service providers control decisions about resource allocation; but undergirding these decisions are definitions and assumptions grounded in professional bodies of knowledge, clinical experience, and the cultures of particular organizational contexts. Care-planning decisions thus reflect the reality of service systems as much as that of clients' needs, and the dependency of clients derives from the pro-fessional paradigms and organizational interests at work.

In response, service recipients may seek independence and control, at-tempting "to establish a reciprocal relationship to mask the dependency so created" (Lloyd, 1991, p. 130). It is these dynamics that can help us under-stand such cases as that of Mr. Valducci, discussed at the beginning of the chapter, in which the client behaves in ways the service system labels *treatment resistant*. The case of Miss Singleton provides further illustration:

Miss Singleton has been a client in the Project since its beginning. A singer on the stage in her youth, she lives alone in an apartment surrounded by records and books she treasures. She has a history of high blood pressure and has been diagnosed as having Organic Brain Syndrome.

Miss Singleton enjoys a daily ride on local public transportation and does her banking in the transit terminal. In the process, she reportedly shows people her money and talks about how much she has. She has been mugged several times after such episodes. The Project has tried unsuccessfully to convince her to have a volunteer service do her banking for her. The Project also referred her to Meals on Wheels, but the service was discontinued after she said she had flushed the meals down the toilet.

The plan at that point became, as a case manager described it, to "put her in a nursing home because she's unsafe." Miss Singleton reportedly agreed with this description of herself and agreed to be put on the waiting list for one of the homes the staff took her to visit, but then balked at going to be interviewed there. The staff then arranged an appointment for her at a geriatric counseling service at which she was "known" (that is, she had been a client there before) in order for the staff there "to talk to her about going to a nursing home." When the nurse arrived to take her to the appointment, she refused to go. The nurse called the service to reschedule the appointment. When Miss Singleton stated she still would not go, the nurse called again, canceling the appointment and saying the client had a cold. Shortly before the rescheduled time, Miss Singleton herself called the service and said she was ready to go, and it was the nurse who didn't feel well.

Clients like Mr. Valducci and Miss Singleton may indeed be offering resistance, but not merely to the specific services proposed as part of a professionally designed care plan. Their resistance takes place on a more global level—that is, to the ways case managers attempt to define and reshape their lives in order to make them more categorically compatible with the requirements of service systems. Miss Singleton's strategies of resistance responded to the hermeneutic nature of this struggle.

Discussion

Because of their positions spanning the boundaries of people-processing organizations, case managers face multiple, competing obligations—to clients, to family members, to their professional knowledge and codes of ethics, and to their own agency and other service providers. Dilemmas they encounter in practice often trace to conflicts of interest embedded in this situation (Clemens et al., 1994). Such conflicts concern the provision of services, but ultimately they are less about what is delivered than about the terms of its delivery: who will define what is needed and how it will be provided.

Sociologist Peter Lloyd (1991, p. 129) notes that debates about community-based care take the form of contrasting discourses about these micropolitical questions:

The consensus discourse assumes that all those who are involved in the assessment of the needs of the elderly person and in assembling the package of care and support services are people of good will, seeing as their prime objective the best and correct solution. They work together in partnership. . . . Technical difficulties, when they occur, can be resolved through amicable discussion.

Such assumptions clearly have guided the rationale and design of case management programs in long-term care. In practice, however, case management appears shaped more by "structural contradictions and conflicts of individual interest," which Lloyd refers to as a contrasting "conflict discourse." Paramount among these conflicts is, as he puts it, "the independence and control sought by the elderly individual which conflicts with the creation of dependency by all those offering care and support" (Lloyd, 1991, p. 130). While this is true for relations with family and other informal caregivers, the structural nature of this conflict is even more apparent within the type of formal care delivery case management represents:

> A bottom-up approach which stresses the right of elderly individuals or consumers to services, to express their needs and have a say in the selection of services offered, to control their delivery and to protest when things go wrong is incompatible [sic] with the top-down approach with management assessing needs and deciding who is most needy, allocating accordingly scarce resources, rationed by a limitation on funding, and adopting a professional stance before the dependent recipient of services. (Lloyd, 1991, p. 129)

Proposals to shift the objectives of case management in long-term care from maintaining people in the community to empowering clients represent one response to this conflict. Adopting the tenets and programs of the independent living movement would be one way to move in this direction. It is unclear, however, how adaptable the independent living model is to the needs of elders, particularly those, like Miss Singleton, with cognitive deficits. Initial research on the appropriateness of the independent living model indicates a lack of clear criteria to evaluate which older clients would be good candidates for consumer-directed home care; using consensus between a case manager and an independent assessor as the standard, less than 20% of a particular home care program's clients would qualify (Scala et al., 1996). Other work suggests that older consumers may not have as strong a preference as younger ones for controlling services (Eustis & Fischer, 1992). Self-directed case management in particular may therefore be less appropriate for them even in a model more generally aimed at consumer direction.

It would not be necessary, however, to adopt a new approach in order to improve the responsiveness of our current long-term care system to consumer perspectives. Surveys show that current long-term care case management programs tend to elicit and respond to client preferences in a haphazard, unsystematic manner. One study of elder services programs in 24 states found few providing extensive guidance to case managers on involving clients in care planning; and the materials used still reflect an assumption of professional control, with little attention to client opinion. Moreover, clients typically receive only limited information about program operations, and grievance procedures, though in existence, are rarely governed by very specific provisions or adequately explained to clients. A second study confirmed that case managers do not view client preferences as having a major impact on care plans (Leutz, Sciegaj, & Capitman, 1997; Kane, Penrod, & Kivnick, 1994).

There is thus much that can be done, even within the present system of care, to increase client empowerment. To do this will, however, require renewed dedication to system change and advocacy on clients' behalf. We will review the prospects for this as we conclude by surveying the present state of case management in long-term care.

CONCLUSION: WHERE WE ARE NOW

The legacy of case management's development in long-term care is a mosaic of programs varying along multiple dimensions: the type of services they provide and the type of organization they are part of; their goals and sources of funding; the extent to which case managers control service resources or engage in direct service provision; the intensity, scope, and duration of case management; and the type of client or target group (Geron & Chassler, 1994). Notwithstanding this variegation, there are, in general, both broad and significant differences between public and private sector case management.

In the public sector, case management remains an integral part of Medicaid, Older Americans Act, and state-funded long-term care programs. State agencies clearly value the use of case management: In a recent survey for the Senate Special Committee on Aging, almost all state Medicaid offices and state agencies on aging ranked case management very useful as a way to determine service needs of disabled elders, second in utility only to a standard assessment instrument or protocol. They further identified case management as one of the services most needed by elderly persons with severe disabilities (USGAO, 1994a).

At the same time, funding for these programs remains an issue of perpetual concern, with clear implications for the role of case managers. State officials in long-term care programs acknowledge that case managers function primarily as gatekeepers to service systems, fulfilling what they deem an essential cost containment role. This has become particularly critical for long-term care community-based programs operating solely with state funds. Older Americans Act funding has also been continuously curtailed, showing appropriations in 1995 roughly half of those of 1973, once adjusted for inflation and demographic growth (USGAO, 1994b; Administration on Aging, 1995).

Specific measures states use to control expenditures include using annual or per-client caps on expenditures (typical for Medicaid programs), rationing and restricting services, establishing waiting lists, increasing the sizes of case managers' caseloads, and reducing the number of case manager positions (USGAO, 1993, 1994b). All of these measures place additional burdens on case managers, in addition to the inherent contradiction between their charge to act as client advocates while curtailing service expenditures. Not surprisingly, case managers experience their gatekeeper and money management functions as sources of role strain and ethical dilemmas (Kane et al., 1994).

In the private sector, especially for health care, case management operates as a form of profit enhancement—a "service line" in itself or a way of ensuring the productivity of other product lines (Satinsky, 1995). This has also become true for nonprofit agencies, which mimic their proprietary counterparts by adopting strategies to enhance their competitiveness: unbundling services for greater reimbursement, eliminating unprofitable services, and increasing client turnover (Estes et al., 1993), all purposes facilitated by case management.

Case management's historical role in enhancing access to services exists now mainly for those who can afford it—as individuals, by purchasing a private case manager's services; for both individuals and organizations, by having the resources to authorize or purchase care above the standard reimbursement; for companies, by purchasing a case management program as part of employee assistance or family care benefits. These abilities, too, largely parallel the line between public and private, since public case management clients remain limited by and to what the state will fund.

At the same time that we have moved toward a two-tier system of case management, the norms and values guiding case management have shifted across the board to subordinate objectives of access and advocacy. Recently, a board of experts, convened as the National Advisory Committee on Long-Term Care Case Management by the Robert Wood Johnson Foundation and charged to "achieve consensus about case management and explore the feasibility of developing case management practice guidelines for long-term care" (Geron & Chassler, 1994, p. 92), summed up the current view of case management as "a consumer-centered, flexible, cost-conscious, and quality-driven service" (Geron & Chassler, 1995, p. 10). Embedded in this description are contradictory principles, recognized in the committee's report by noting that "inherent tensions exist between case management's competing responsibilities to consumers and payers" as case management has become "a cost-conscious service that operates within a context of payer requirements and limitations" (Ibid.). While these experts (many of whom had previous involvement with community care demonstrations) are apparently neutral about how such tensions should be resolved, their guidelines for long-term care case management contain such telling statements as the following:

> Within the context of payer requirements, case managers should endeavor to determine and strive to honor the values and preferences of the consumer in all phases of practice. . . . Consumers will need to be informed that in some programs payer requirements specify that receipt of case management monitoring and oversight is a condition of receiving provider services. (Geron & Chassler, 1995, pp. 11–12)

This perspective normalizes the immutability of "payer requirements" while making "consumer-centered" aspects secondary to or derivative of what can be done within the current program context. Advocacy and access, fundamental goals for earlier programs even if counterbalanced by cost containment objectives, practically drop from view in this formulation. Indeed, the committee agreed, on reviewing the literature on case management function, that advocacy is not an "essential function" that "must be present before the services can be described as case management," but is instead a service "that case managers perform with more or less frequency given the particular context in which the case management is provided" (Geron & Chassler, 1994, p. 96).

Countering this emphasis are calls for consumer-directed programs, particularly ones based on the independent living model. This movement is, however, barely underway and moving against the weight of an entrenched paradigm of provider-directed case management, with the client in a more passive role (Batavia et al., 1991; Sabatino & Litvak, 1992).

Less than 50 years from now, America will have an older population larger than its entire population a century ago (Treas, 1995). At the same time, the elderly will have become more diverse in racial and ethnic background, with a majority projected to come from other than Anglo or European backgrounds by the year 2080 (Torres-Gil, 1992). These trends add urgency to our efforts to shape systems of care that are suitable, effective, and affordable. Although it may not be clear what the face or place of case management will be in this broader effort, because it has become an essential service technology, there will certainly be case management. The increasing numbers and diversity of our aging population argue, as well, that advocacy, access, and consumer direction take front seats as goals for case management in long-term care. If they do not, we run the risk of reinforcing the very inequalities and inadequacies in our service systems that case managers daily struggle to overcome.

NOTES

1. The term *long-term care* refers to a "spectrum of medical, personal, and social services provided to aged and disabled individuals because of diminished capacity for self-care" (Rabin & Stockton, 1987, p. v). Community-based long-term care encompasses a wide scope of service provision, including home care, day care, respite care, nutrition and home-delivered meal programs, geriatric assessment units, hospice care, mental health programs, protective social services, housing services, adult foster care, transportation, telephone reassurance, and emergency alarm service (Kane & Kane, 1987). The focus of this chapter is on demonstration programs using case management to coordinate home care and other supportive programs delivering care to elderly people deemed at risk of nursing home admission.
2. It should also be noted that case management of community-based care here did not arrive de novo, but owed much to earlier programs. In the mid-1950s, the National Commission on Chronic Illness had put forward the concept of coordinating expanded services for individuals with multiple, long-term care needs (Vogel & Palmer, 1985). By the early 1970s, many programs nationwide had already developed comprehensive care approaches to home care that included homemaker and social services as well as medical care; the project run by Montefiore Hospital in New York drew special attention as a program standard (Benjamin, 1993).
3. Rochefort (1986) describes a variety of studies from the 1950s and 1960s showing negative, stereotypic attitudes and beliefs regarding the aged, albeit with mixed findings and validity issues that complicate interpretation. In contrast, however, almost uniformly positive views emerged from a 1974 Lou Harris and Associates survey focused on public perceptions regarding old age; for example, 74% of respondents agreed that older people were very "friendly and warm," and 79% that "there is a real need for people to join together to work toward improving the conditions and social status of people over sixty-five in this country" (Ibid., p. 77). These attitudes translated, in turn, into positive opinions about public support for policies and programs targeted to the aged.
4. For example, witnesses at the reauthorization hearings held before the Subcommittee on Aging of the Senate Committee on Human Resources included representatives of state, county, and city offices on aging; state and area agencies on aging; the Federal Council on Aging; the National Caucus on the Black Aged; National Indian Council on the Aging; Asociacion Nacional Pro Personas Mayores; Meals-on-Wheels and other nutrition projects; American Association of Retired Persons (AARP); Gray Panthers; American Association of Homes for the Aging; and a variety of other com-

munity, academic, and professional agencies (Subcommittee on Aging 1978).

5. Ironically, support for nursing home care had originally come from claims that it would provide a cost-effective substitute for hospital care; cf. White House Conference, 1961.

6. Features commonly waived included eligibility requirements, aspects of benefits, and stipulations that programs be offered statewide. Projects also relied on regular Medicare and Medicaid reimbursements, state and local service agency funding, and service resources made available through the Older Americans Act.

7. ACCESS, for instance, secured friendly visiting, transportation, housing improvement, home maintenance, help with heavy chores, housing and moving assistance, and respite care.

8. These, in turn, were among broader demonstrations around the turn of this decade involving programs as diverse as adult care, home health care, mental health care, and alternative reimbursement for nursing homes. These demonstrations held common objectives designed to rationalize and economize health care delivery. (See Vogel & Palmer, 1985.)

9. At the 1980 APHA meetings, for example, several sessions on community care featured presentations on issues in planning, design, implementation, and evaluation of such programs. Georgia's Health Alternative Services program, Triage, and Nursing Home Without Walls were early case management programs represented by presenters, as were home care, homemaker, and day care programs, and agencies on aging (American Public Health Association, 1980).

10. Delegates on the committee proposing that recommendation (the Technical Committee on Social and Health Aspects of Long Term Care) included executive-level representatives of On Lok and Triage, state and local departments and councils on aging, an American Medical Association committee on long-term care, and service provider agencies and nursing homes; in short, a clear representation of the aging enterprise.

11. Studies also shed little light on an issue newly of policy concern, namely, the impact of these programs on family members caring for an elderly relative. Great concern had arisen, especially within more conservative political circles, that community care and similar programs would undermine support by family caregivers, substituting public dollars for family responsibility (Barusch, 1991). Program advocates countered that instead of this "substitution effect," programs would help expand family efforts by making sure caregivers were not overburdened. An overall evaluation found mixed evidence: While community care programs seemed to substitute for some caregiver assistance with everyday tasks, they did not otherwise seem to affect informal caregivers either by replacing them or by extending their capacities (Kemper et al., 1987).

12. This was true across sites as well as within subgroups categorized according to various indicators of vulnerability, such as disability level, living arrangements, and Medicaid eligibility.

13. Neither model had an impact on performance of Instrumental Activities of

Daily Living, and there was no impact on Activities of Daily Living (ADL) in the Basic model. The Financial Control model clients showed a puzzling decrease in their ability to perform ADL tasks without assistance; this may have been a measuring artifact related to the fact that clients were increasingly receiving such assistance.

14. Findings regarding nursing home utilization may reflect Medicaid reimbursement policies that, by this point, had constrained nursing home bed supplies as well as expenditures, making cost-effective substitution of community care for nursing home use more difficult to achieve (Kemper, 1988; Applebaum & Austin, 1990). Some other methodological issues related to more subtle aspects of program dynamics. Despite the fact that this project studied case management more systematically than had been done before, its measure of the receipt of such services still consisted of "yes/no" scales. There was no way to evaluate the intensity of case management in either model (that is, the extent to which case managers were actively engaged with clients and advocated on their behalf) or to assess the quality of care plans, client compliance, or direct services (Kane, 1988).

15. I studied the Project for an 18-month period using participant observation and informal interviews to examine case managers' activities, views of clients, and working relations with other agencies. All names given here are pseudonyms, and identifying personal attributes have been altered to preserve confidentiality.

3

Case Management for People With Chronic Mental Illness

Institutions Without Walls

The Community Mental Health Centers Act of 1963 launched what the director of the National Institute of Mental Health termed "one of the most dynamic revolutions in the history of the mental health movement" (Rochefort, 1986, p. 25). The main thrust of this revolution was the release of thousands of individuals from state psychiatric institutions, permanently transforming where and how services would be provided for people with severe and chronic mental illness.[1] These changes introduced new demands on service providers to respond to the needs of former patients— needs for housing, employment, social activity, health care, and all the other hallmarks of living in a noninstitutional setting. In essence, the mental health service system needed to recreate the institution, but without its walls or restrictions.

Case management emerged in response to this need. The developers of case management promoted it as a way to support people in the community by increasing their access to comprehensive, coordinated sources of care. Over the next decades, case management would become mandated as a standard feature of mental health programs and a cornerstone of both simple and ambitious attempts to overhaul the mental health sector.

This chapter examines the broad antecedents and the specific history of mental health case management. First, we seek its origins in the dilemmas that followed the revolution of deinstitutionalization. Then, we trace its chronological development as different approaches mirrored the broader policy issues of their times. As in long-term care, we will see over time a shift in the objectives of case management programs, from being gate-keepers to increase clients' access to services, to using such gatekeeping as part of extensive cost containment efforts. While this introduces particular strains into case managers' roles, case management practice has always embodied diverse and contradictory objectives because it attempts to address the needs of the mental health system as well as those of service recipients. We will also see that there are still many barriers to the ability of individuals with serious mental illness to live satisfying, independent lives, barriers to some extent created by the limitations of the service system itself. In these respects, case management, itself an institution without walls, operates within contexts where the walls are less visible, but no less concrete than the walls of the asylum. In the final section, we examine how case management practice embodies these contradictions and tensions of the broader service system.

"BETTER BUT NOT WELL": MENTAL HEALTH CARE IN THE AFTERMATH OF DEINSTITUTIONALIZATION

The Failures of Community Care

Mental health case management has dual roots in the deinstitutionalization movement of the 1960s. On the one hand, policies and programs within the movement included services similar to what would become case management and providers with responsibilities like case managers. Changes at this time in the overall system of mental health care as well as its clients also furthered the move toward case management. On the other hand, it was the failures of deinstitutionalization that convinced mental health providers of the need for better ways to support people with chronic mental illness in the community, a need case management would be designed to meet.

Many interests and forces supported the movement to remove people with chronic mental illness from state hospitals and treat them in community settings.[2] State and federal policies favoring deinstitutionalization had deeper roots in the socioenvironmental and psychotherapeutic orientations of psychiatry following World War II (see Gronfein, 1985; Brown, 1985; Rosen, Pancake, & Rickards, 1995). The National Institute of Mental Health had advocated for community-based services since the mid-1940s. Institutional care had come under blistering academic and media criticism. New drugs reducing psychiatric symptoms made care in the community seem increasingly viable. Federal entitlement and disability programs shifted the burden of sustaining community care to deeper pockets than those of state and local providers. One such program, Medicaid, initially spawned the "transinstitutionalization" of patients from mental hospital to nursing home settings (Gronfein, 1985; Brown, 1985) but would ultimately support a range of community care options.

While scholars differ in their assessment of the importance of these different features in promoting deinstitutionalization policy,[3] most acknowledge the role of changing modes and structures of care supported by new social, professional, and policy perspectives on mental illness. Case management would emerge bolstered by these views and structures.

One key philosophical underpinning of deinstitutionalization was the concept of the community as a therapeutic environment; that is, the idea that living in the community could foster healthy behavior, social support and integration, and life skills for hospital patients who were "better but not well" (Klerman, 1977, p. 628; cf. Thompson, Griffith, & Leaf, 1990; Mechanic, 1986; Rochefort, 1997). Within the first decade following the Community Mental Health Centers Act (the federal salvo of deinstitutionalization), it was apparent to mental health leaders and policymakers alike that living in the community was anything but therapeutic for these individuals. The President's Commission on Mental Health, established in 1977 to evaluate the mental health care system, pronounced:

> Time and again we have learned—from testimony, from inquiries, and from the reports of special task panels—of people with chronic mental disabilities who have been released from hospitals but who do not have the basic necessities of life. They lack adequate food, clothing, or shelter. We have heard of woefully inadequate follow-up mental health and general medical care. And we have seen evidence that half the people released from large mental hospitals are being readmitted within a year of discharge. While not every individual can be treated within the community, many of the readmissions to State hospitals could have been avoided if comprehensive assistance had existed within their communities. (The President's Commission on Mental Health, vol. 1, 1978, p. 5)

Gaps in care, fragmentation of services, lack of continuity and follow-up, and the absence of the "basic necessities" were widely decried in journalistic, professional, and governmental venues as a "national disgrace" (Reich, 1973; U.S. General Accounting Office, 1977; Turner & TenHoor, 1978; Chu & Trotter, 1974). What had gone wrong? Most analysts pointed to insufficient supply and coordination of the diverse support services needed to maintain people within the community. Inadequacies in the number of community mental health centers and in their attention to clients with chronic mental illness were additional problems (The President's Commission, op. cit; Bachrach, 1976; Reich, 1973; Becker & Schulberg, 1976; Stein & Test, 1978; Test & Stein, 1976).

It would take more than services and funding dollars to transform a system centered on institutional care. Also needed were ways to re-create the diverse functions performed by the mental hospital, such as providing for such essentials as food, housing, and hygiene and coordinating psychological, social, medical and custodial care. Rather than receiving these through community agencies, many former patients were "transinstitutionalized," placed in nursing homes, board and care facilities, or single-room occupancy hotels that often became "psychiatric ghettos" where residents received little care, or care worse than that of state facilities (Burt & Pittman, 1985, p. 68; cf. Aviram & Segal, 1973; Brown, 1985). In addition, community-based service providers were neither trained nor inclined to treat a population that was considered incurable, that had extensive psychosocial needs, and that would not respond well to usual modes of treatment (Johnson & Rubin, 1983; Stein & Test, 1978). In short, there was a lack of a conceptual framework for a new system of care as well as the infrastructure to make it happen (Thompson et al., 1990; Mechanic, 1986).

At the same time that criticism of community care rose, states continued to follow a policy of deinstitutionalization. In part this followed financial incentives (particularly for nursing home placements, which were federally subsidized through Medicaid) and the clinical ability to control symptoms with newer drugs (Rochefort, 1997; Rosen et al., 1995). The policy trend also, however, relied on the continued belief that care in the community was better than that in the hospital. Backing this viewpoint was the proposition that institutionalization, even for a short-term stay, created a dependency in patients and their families that led to a "revolving door" of recidivism (Thompson et al., 1990). While the mental hospital was generally acknowledged as a necessary of the overall treatment system, even those who acknowledged the hospital's value as a place where people who could not cope would be safe—an "asylum" in every sense (Lamb, 1986)—wanted its use minimized (Bachrach, 1976; Harris, Bergman, & Greenwood, 1982). By the mid-1970s, three-quarters of persons receiving formal mental health care did so on an outpatient basis, and the estimated census of state mental hospitals in 1975 was less than 200,000, down from 550,000 twenty years earlier (The President's Commission on Mental Illness, vol. 1, 1978).

These changes in services occurred in the context of major shifts in the structure and financing of the overall system of mental health care, shifts that accompanied a move from state to federal funding. Before 1960, mental health services were almost exclusively the province of states, both financially and administratively. Under the Community Mental Health Centers Act, federal funding bypassed the state mental health agencies that administered state hospitals, going instead directly to community mental health centers. Medicaid was a second source of federal financing replacing, in part, state expenditures. As noted, many Medicaid dollars went to inpatient care (either in nursing homes and intermediate care facilities or general or state psychiatric hospitals), but Medicaid also covered psychotropic medication costs and medical and dental care in addition to mental health services for people with chronic mental illness in the community. Supplemental Security Income, enacted in 1974, was a third source of federal funding that directly contributed to maintaining people with disabling mental illness in the community.

Although the extent of federal leadership in mental health care would shortly plummet relative to the early days of deinstitutionalization, much of the financing structure created by the mid-1970s remains in place today, with lasting consequences for mental health services and their clients. Because of this structure, the sector started to change from public to private auspices in two ways. First, proprietary services (nursing homes and board and care facilities, in particular) emerged to capture Medicaid funding and SSI dollars. Second, in the nonprofit sector, agencies began to rely on contract funding under community mental health center (CMHC) and Medicaid initiatives, a change that would expand into a "contracting regime" under block grants (Smith & Lipsky, 1993). The impact on people with serious mental illness was equally pronounced. They now had to connect not just with different providers but with totally different programs to piece together their livelihood, living arrangements, and medical and psychiatric care. Additionally, every program was part of a different bureaucratic system, each with its own criteria, standards, and procedures. As means-tested programs, SSI and Medicaid bore the stigma and vulnerability of the welfare sector, adding to that already experienced by people with serious mental illness.

New Patients and Consumers

Along with changes in the way care was delivered came a new type of care recipient: young adults with chronic mental illness who had little history of institutional care. The terms describing this population in the literature reveal the conflation of their problems with those of the service system: "the young adult chronic patient"; "treatment resisters"; or "acute care recidivists" (Pepper, Kirshner, & Ryglewicz, 1981; Goldfinger, Hopkin, & Surber, 1984). All denoted individuals with "severe difficulties in social functioning, and [a] tendency to use mental health services inappropriately, in ways that drain the time and energy of clinicians yet do not conform to viable treatment plans" (Pepper et al., 1981, p. 463). Unlike the older, initial deinstitutionalized patient, these individuals were of working age (roughly 18 to 40) and had frequent but brief stays in inpatient facilities in addition to high levels of use of a range of outpatient, emergency, and residential services (Goldfinger et al., 1984; Caton, 1981). While some had adapted to a patient role through initial hospitalization at a young age, more common was resistance to the label and identity of being mentally ill, accompanied by sporadic adherence to treatment plans and drug regimens. Clinical discussions pointed to their personal failures, impulsive and manipulative behavior, alcohol and substance abuse, poor judgment, and attribution of blame to external forces (including their mental health providers) as factors that made the "young chronics" unlike older patients and harder to treat (Sheets, Prevost, & Reihman, 1982; Pepper et al., 1981; cf. Pepper & Ryglewicz, 1982).

Mental health providers saw this group as posing multiple challenges to the system, even as they acknowledged that the system was failing to address the group's needs. Lack of services and of clinical contact, continuity, and coordination were especially problematic for individuals like these with multiple types of needs (Goldfinger et al., 1984). An implicit assumption was that these were people worth trying to return to adult functioning, and in particular some form of vocation. However, even more basic services were often lacking and vocational ones were not well connected with the rest of the system. Moreover, what the system could offer was often not meaningful to these young adults, for many of whom basic housing and subsistence needs weighed heavier than therapeutic goals (Ibid; Hopper, Baxter, & Cox, 1982).

While this group of clients challenged the professional authority of psychiatry in a particular way, there were broader objections to the professional domination of mental health care. Civil actions from the mid-1960s to the late 1970s redefined the legal rights of mental health recipients, including procedural safeguards in involuntary commitment, the right to the "least restrictive setting" of care, and the rights to receive as well as to refuse treatment (LaFond & Durham, 1992; Friedman & Yohalem, 1978; Chandler, 1990). As in the broader field of health care, there was increased emphasis on the "consumer" voice of care recipients and on the need for consumer advocates within the system (Brown, 1985).

Beyond specific implications for treatment, both the new patients and the consumer movement demanded a new level of responsiveness from the mental health system. Policymakers and program planners sought ways to provide connection to and coordination of the varied services needed to sustain community living; they also recognized the need for a personal therapeutic relationship to sustain that connection on a long-term basis (Goldfinger et al., 1984).

New Roles for Old and New Staff

One obvious and essential time for an individual with mental illness to start making connections to the community was during discharge from a psychiatric hospital. In the late 1960s, some state hospitals began providing intensive follow-up in communities. Describing efforts that would later become the Program for Assertive Community Treatment, one of the most widely adopted treatment models, Thompson et al. (1990, p. 626) observe that "Ward staff visited patients at home, worked closely with patients' social networks, and were available almost around the clock to help with problems in living." Other programs used paraprofessionals in community agencies, including mental health centers, to help patients bridge to aftercare and as "expediters" to maintain service rosters and facilitate referrals for clients (Alley, Blanton, & Feldman, 1979; Platman, Dorgan, Gerhard, Mallam, & Spiliadis, 1982; Reif & Reissman, 1965). By the end of the 1960s, there was graduate training for this role, which had broadened to provide assessment, planning, monitoring, support, and advocacy (Hansell, Wodarczyk, & Visotsky, 1968; Granet & Talbott, 1978; cf. Platman et al., 1982; Levine, Tulkin, Intagliata, Perry, & Whitson, 1979).

Clearly the prototypes for mental health case management, these new roles emerged as part of a broader effort to provide training and job services for workers in the burgeoning human service sector that followed Great Society initiatives. To a large extent, employment in the human services opened up nonprofessional positions aimed at "indigenous" workers, who were disproportionately minority group members with low job skills (Reif & Reissman, 1965). Exemplifying the momentum of this movement, by 1976, workers with less than a bachelor's degree made up over 50% of service personnel in a national survey of mental health facilities (James, 1979). Mental health nonprofessionals staffed services ranging from more administrative functions such as intake to distinctly clinical ones, such as individual and group counseling (Sobey, 1970).

While it is not clear how many of these new workers had been staff in state hospitals, the future of hospital workers was of great concern as deinstitutionalization progressed. As state employees, many staff were union members represented by the American Federation of State, County and Municipal Employees (AFSCME). AFSCME was vocal on their needs, advocating their right to transfer to community facilities and receive retraining at state expense (Perlman, 1976). These issues also clearly shaped the judgments by the President's Commission on Mental Health; this commission's Task Panel reporting on deinsitutionalization, rehabilitation, and long-term care (1978, p. 366) recommended that "The Federal Government ensure funds for the training and retraining of professionals and paraprofessionals who wish to care for the chronically mentally disabled and promote a National policy for career advancement in this special field."

Even before such funds became available, the division of labor in the mental health field had changed dramatically. Following the Community Mental Health Care Act, psychologists and social workers filled new clinical positions in community mental health centers, and the expansion of both their ranks and the scope of their expertise challenged the dominance of psychiatrists (James, 1979; Brown, 1985). By the mid-1970s, the most rapidly growing categories of mental health workers were, however, other professional workers (those with a bachelor's degree or higher level of education) and paraprofessionals (those with less than a bachelor's degree) engaged in patient care.

While some experts worried that nonprofessionals were taking over professional jobs and others were concerned that they were handling only menial responsibilities, there was not necessarily a clear difference between the roles of professional and paraprofessional workers in mental health centers. This was particularly apparent for some of the tasks that would later typify case management. For example, a 1970 survey of National Institute of Mental Health–funded programs found that the task of facilitating access to community services was equally divided between nonprofessional and professional workers (Sobey, 1970). More generally, nonprofessionals appeared to take on new roles and to serve groups professionals had not reached, such as poorer clients.

By the end of the 1970s, the human resources of the mental health care system looked as different from the picture presented at the beginning of the decade as did the service setting. With community-based care came a host of new positions. While some were based on traditional, clinical functions, others related to perceptions that ex-patients needed help living in the community and connecting with the resources required to stay there.

Reinforcing Community Supports

A decade and a half after community mental health care was legislated into existence, the provision of care for people with chronic mental illness was in some respects less secure than it had been under the old state hospital system. To get services and even the basic necessities, clients now had to connect with a variety of service systems and providers. New cohorts of clients were disadvantaged by homelessness and characteristics, such as substance abuse, that led providers to see them as more difficult and less desirable service recipients.[4] Further increasing their vulnerability was their dependence on social welfare programs such as SSI and Medicaid, which were themselves vulnerable to cutbacks.

Mental health leaders had not given up on the community, however. Critiques of deinstitutionalization targeted service system fragmentation as a major flaw undermining community-based care. A leading analyst outlined the resulting belief that "most of the problems of deinstitutionalization could be resolved if there were a concerted effort to improve coordination at the federal, state, and local level among the various health and social agencies that serve the chronically mentally ill" (Lamb, 1981, p. 105). While there was increased acceptance that some hospitalization was an inevitable, or even desirable, part of the system, the major thrust of social policy for the next decade and a half would be to bolster community care through program innovations focused on service integration. The first of these, the Community Support Program of 1977, would also be the first formal mandate for mental health case management.

THE HEART OF COMMUNITY SUPPORT: CASE MANAGEMENT COMES OF AGE

With shifts from state to federal funding, from the mental health system to the welfare system, and from the public to the proprietary sector, responsibility for the organizing and financing of care for people with serious mental illness had become fragmented and confused. The National Institute of Mental Health, which lacked formal authority over service providers and provided only limited funding, nonetheless began to assume a leadership role in designing a model promoting comprehensive, coordinated services at both the state and local level. In 1974, Dr. Lucy Ozarin convened an ad hoc internal Community Support Work Group within NIMH; over the next three years, this group would encompass representatives from all divisions of NIMH as well as other Department of Health, Education, and Welfare (HEW) offices and federal agencies. Working conferences involved state mental health, welfare, and Medicaid representatives in defining the concept of community support systems and identifying implementation strategies. In 1978, NIMH awarded the first Community Support Program (CSP) contracts to 19 states to develop service planning as well as demonstration programs.[5] The goal of CSP was to foster "community support systems" (CSSs), which NIMH guidelines defined as "a network of caring and responsible people committed to assisting a vulnerable population to meet their needs and develop their potentials without being unnecessarily isolated or excluded from the community" (Turner & TenHoor, 1978, p. 329). Operationally, the CSSs took the form of organizational arrangements coordinating different community programs and service providers. CSP contracts required that a core services agency either provide or subcontract for comprehensive assessment of needs and guarantee the legislative, administrative, and financial arrangements necessary to meet those needs. Part of this guarantee involved identifying *"a single person (or team)* at the client level *responsible* for remaining in touch with the client on a continuing basis, regardless of how many agencies get involved" (CSP RFPs 1977, cited in Turner & TenHoor, 1978, p. 330, italics in original). This person or team was, of course, the case manager. Although it was not clear which agency, or even which sector, would assume responsibility for case management, NIMH specifically required it as one of 10 essential clinical and administrative CSS components.

The CSP program sought not to support direct services, but to stimulate state planning and promote local-level CSS demonstrations. Modest in funding, the program nonetheless rapidly widened its scope, such that by the 1984 fiscal year it provided grant support to all 50 states, the District of Columbia, and 2 territories. The concept of the CSS was at least as important as the actual programs initiated, however, since it marked the mental health sector's claim to leadership in taking responsibility for an array of rehabilitation and support services in addition to its own. To this day, the community support system concept remains a model dominating discussions of state and local mental health system planning.

The case management model embedded in CSP closely resembled the role of case manager previously developed in the Balanced Service System (BSS) program used by the Joint Commission on Accreditation of Hospitals as its source for accreditation standards for community mental health centers.[6] The BSS case manager was a "human service generalist" who ensured continuity of care for clients across all service systems through assessment, planning, linking, monitoring, and advocacy activities (Sullivan, 1981; Dorgan & Gerhard, 1979; Cohen & Devine, 1979). Case managers could be professionals as well as paraprofessional workers, but the emphasis was on their service integration and monitoring functions, not direct clinical care. A description of an "aftercare program" in Cambridge, Massachusetts, in 1979 provides a good sense of the case manager's role:

> Prior to their discharge from the state hospitals, patients are helped by their paraprofessional case manager to assess their own needs. In addition, before clients leave the hospital, the paraprofessionals take them on community visits for familiarization with grocery shopping, choice of housing, and other matters important in community transition. After clients are discharged, the paraprofessionals help them in many matters, including disputes with welfare or landlords, arrangement for placement in a vocational rehabilitation program, and consultation with personnel of a community day-care facility attended by the client. In several instances, the paraprofessionals have created new programs . . . to fill needs otherwise unmet by existing resources. (Cohen & Devine, 1979, p. 218)

Case management was so central to CSS operations that an official from the Michigan Department of Mental Health declared at an NIMH conference, "We view the heart of CSP as case management. We're looking for a case-management system that the State can build CSP around and into" (National Institute of Mental Health, 1982, p. 112). Case managers were equally central to service delivery. One early evaluation of CSP found that for most services received by clients, a case manager was in some way involved over 80% of the time (Tessler, Goldman, & Associates, 1982).

A Paradoxical Assortment

There was, however, little uniformity either in the structure of case management or in the requirements of case managers. For the most part, states assigned case management to existing staff. While there was some criticism of this as simply a new way to exploit federal funding,[7] states countered that they could not afford to create new, independent case management systems. CSS case managers thus worked in a variety of programs. Lead agencies for CSSs themselves varied in their organizational site and responsibilities. While some were state psychiatric facilities, others were regional mental health authorities, community-based mental health providers, or broader social service programs. Some lead agencies subcontracted for direct services and provided mainly coordination; others supplied all direct services. In addition, different departments or providers within the CSS could offer their own type of case management, focused on the specific needs of their clients (Grusky et al., 1986; Love, 1984).

The contexts in which case management occurred also became more variable as CSP funding fueled the expansion of several types of programs in the community. Two of the most often replicated of these were the psychosocial rehabilitation model associated with Fountain House, a "clubhouse" program in which professional staff and "members" aimed for interdependent, less hierarchical relations; and the Training in Community Living model (TCL, with the service component named the Program of Assertive Community Treatment, or PACT), in which interdisciplinary service teams providing assertive outreach and individualized treatment focused on community living skills (Stroul, 1986). Just as programs varied in their treatment philosophies, in the range of services commanded for clients, and in the degree to which they connected with client's family members and other "natural supports," so too did different models of case management (Pescosolido, Wright, & Sullivan, 1995; Rapp & Kisthardt, 1996).

The caseloads, roles, and characteristics of case managers varied accordingly. For example, a statewide survey of New York CSS case managers found that they had an average number of clients ranging from 20 to 80 cases and that case managers in voluntary agencies differed from those employed by the state in their age, education, and employment history (McGreevy, 1986). While some CSS sites retained the expediter model, with case managers acting mainly as service brokers, a 1980 survey of over 200 CSP case managers found three-fifths with job titles such as "therapist," "psychologist," "counselor," or "social worker," all suggesting a direct clinical service role (Love, 1984). Similarly, several studies of case managers' time allocation found "face-to-face" direct service activities taking up substantial portions (one-fifth to one-third) of case managers' time, albeit equal or greater amounts of time went to recordkeeping and administrative meetings (Curry, 1980).

The diversity of case management practices reflected a broader lack of clarity about what case management was or should be. Writing from a social work perspective in the early 1980s, Johnson and Rubin noted,

> Despite its growing popularity, case management is still in the early stages of development as a practice model. A major problem is its lack of operational clarity. Its functions have been interpreted in disparate ways, making case management a paradoxical assortment of activities requiring substantial commitment from all organizational levels for successful implementation." (1983, p. 49)

Comparing mental health case managers with those in other settings, researchers found the former reported the least clear understanding about their roles as well as the lowest sense of professional investment in case management per se (Johnson & Rubin, op. cit.). Clients, too, shared the confusion about what to expect from their case managers: A study of a CSS in Alabama found that few clients were aware of the types of help case managers could provide, or even of the existence of CSP case management services as formal entities, even though they were positive about things their own case managers had done for them (Grusky et al., 1986).

One of the biggest areas of both uncertainty and controversy among mental health professionals was the extent to which case managers should be therapeutic agents. Some programs deliberately kept case managers as service brokers, arguing that they would be better able to advocate for clients if located independently of direct service provision (Ibid.). Opposing this position, Richard Lamb, a psychiatrist and leading mental health analyst, felt that while the case manager need not be the primary therapist, case management was inseparable from the therapeutic role. The most meaningful psychotherapy, in Lamb's view, focused on that which was also the essential subject of case management, "the realities and day-to-day issues of life and survival in the community" (Lamb, 1980, p. 763). Echoing this view, another leading commentator testifying at an NIMH conference on CSP referred to a "traveling companion" model of case management, one centered on the survival needs of clients and their relationships with case managers. This role was impossible to perform from behind a desk, he noted, commenting more cynically, "case management is a new group of workers whose job it is to protect the therapists from having to venture

outside the office and deal with the real world's economic issues and problems" (National Institute of Mental Health, 1982, p. 118; cf. Deitchman,
1980).

As the comment reveals, part of the reason the therapeutic role of case
managers was a contentious issue was that the division of labor and control within the mental health sector was itself unsettled. Psychiatry continued to be challenged on professional and ideological grounds, while
psychologists and social workers continued to expand their domains.
Turning over control of cases to paraprofessionals was threatening in some
respects to all, but especially to social workers, whose casework approach
was close to case management both conceptually and in practice (Johnson
& Rubin, 1983).

In the end, however, the questions of who would do case management
and how it would be done were answered by practical contingencies as
much as professional claims. In some states the job market for therapists
declined along with the economy of the late 1970s, so that even paraprofessional case management positions were filled by professional MSWs
(National Institute of Mental Health, 1982). On average, nationally, CSS
case managers had advanced degrees and extensive experience in mental
health care (Bernstein, 1981; Love, 1984). Individual agency policies and
practices influenced what case managers did for clients, and the range of
services clients received varied with that offered by the agency (Korr &
Cloninger, 1991). At the same time, case managers, especially those who
were social workers, tended to drift toward therapeutic activities and relationships with clients. One-on-one work with clients occupied a substantial portion of case managers' time, and much of that appeared to
involve short-term counseling (Curry, 1980). Studies of social workers in
mental health settings found them assigning less importance to brokerage
and advocacy activities than to psychotherapeutic ones. Advocacy in particular seemed short-changed, consistently getting less than 10% of case
managers' time (Curry, 1980; Johnson & Rubin, 1983). Bureaucratic and administrative time demands appeared to be one source of role conflict for
more therapeutically inclined case managers, and turnover in case management staff was reportedly high (Intagliata & Baker, 1983).

Doing More With Less: Case Management
Shifts Its Focus

Five years after its beginnings, it was clear that the CSP approach had not
achieved a large-scale solution to the problems of community mental
health care (Love, 1984). The federal contribution had become limited both
programmatically and financially; at the state level, the stringent economic climate of the late 1970s and early 1980s restrained the expansion of ser-

vices and the replication of CSS demonstration models. The demise of up to half the CSP offices was forecast once federal funding ceased. At both federal and state levels, the focus had been on system integration and interagency collaboration, strategies that made limited fiscal demands but offered equally limited potential for system change. The realities of fiscal and social policy limitations were reflected in the way NIMH now defined the role of case management. While initial program statements emphasized "ensur[ing] continuous availability of appropriate forms of assistance" (Turner & TenHoor, 1978, p. 330), by 1980 the role had become that of a "'resource manager' who . . . can assist the client in coordinating services" (Stroul, 1984, p. 11).

The policy climate of the next decade would ensure that case management retained its place as a central element of mental health care, but with increasing emphasis on goals of cost-effectiveness and service efficiency. The Reagan administration ushered in an era of federal retrenchment, devolving responsibility and authority for human services to the states, which in turn handed it over to local governments. One mechanism for this practice was through block grants, which combined the funding for multiple categorical programs into bigger packages delivered to states with fewer administrative regulations and requirements. Under the Omnibus Budget Reconciliation Act (OBRA) of 1981, mental health service dollars, formerly allocated directly to community mental health centers (CMHCs) and other providers, became part of the alcohol, drug abuse, and mental health services (ADAMH) block grant. At the same time, Congress cut the appropriations for block grant programs, convinced that state-level administration would be more efficient than federal management of categorical programs. These cuts would continue, and ADAMH funding would show a 30.7% decline, in constant dollars, between fiscal 1981 and fiscal 1988. Until now the cornerstone of mental health care in the community, CMHCs were particularly hard hit with revenue losses not made up by states, suffering a decrease of 37% in federal-state support between 1981 and 1983 alone (Rochefort, 1993).[8]

One response by both states and providers was to attempt to garner more funds through other programs, especially Medicaid. Here, federal initiatives both helped and hindered. Simultaneous with block grants, the Reagan administration began tightening eligibility for Supplemental Security Income (SSI) and other income maintenance programs (Burt & Pittman, 1985). Many of those removed from the rolls were people with chronic mental illness who depended on federal support for income and for the access to Medicaid that came with SSI. In addition, OBRA reduced the federal dollars matching state Medicaid expenditures.

OBRA also, however, initiated Medicaid waivers for the primary care case management (PCCM) program, through which states could achieve cost savings by restricting recipients to designated providers. The program also increased Medicaid reimbursement for some services, in particular, case management. From ground zero in 1981, Medicaid case management programs expanded rapidly, enrolling over 651,000 recipients by 1986 (Spitz, 1987). The Consolidated Omnibus Reconciliation Act (COBRA) of 1985 gave case management a further boost by reimbursing it as an "optional" Medicaid service not requiring a federal waiver. Although these programs did not enroll all Medicaid recipients with serious mental health needs,[9] they did augment state mental health dollars. More critically, PCCM linked mental health case management to objectives of cost-effectiveness and efficiency more explicitly than before and tied it to a structure of service delivery that would ultimately be called *managed care*.

Even as other types of mental health service dried up through the 1980s, case management continued to expand. Beyond specific program initiatives like PCCM, case management appears to have offered adaptive advantages to providers forced to adopt a business model of service delivery: one seeking more efficient procedures, higher staff productivity, tighter screening and monitoring of patients and services, and controls on more expensive program stays (Rochefort, 1993, p. 89). Case management staff were among the few personnel additions in CMHCs, consistent with these new practices and with the heightened priority state mental health authorities placed on community services for the chronic mentally ill. Ironically, one study evaluating the extent of fragmentation and duplication in state mental health services in the mid-1980s found that case management was the only service program showing signs of redundancy (Solomon, Gordon, & Davis, 1986).

It was, however, a different form of case management than that envisioned in CSP. Its aims differed in emphasis and, in PCCM, in kind. Case managers were also doing more with less: more searching for ways to provide services or reinstate eligibility for clients; more work with higher caseloads; less service resources for clients; less financial resources for their agencies (Rochefort, 1993; Burt & Pittman, 1985). At the same time, demands for mental health care increased, particularly in areas hardest hit by economic distress.[10] Yet the service levels CMHCs could attain tended to remain stable or even fell as service demands rose (Rochefort, 1993). Trying to cover the most critical junctures of care, some providers converted their case managers to "placement" specialists focused solely on transitions from inpatient to community care. Others moved all "specialist" case managers, who dealt either with specific client populations or types of services, into "generalist" modes. Responding to challenges from the growing mental health consumer movement, some providers trained consumers to be peer case managers (Carling, 1995), and the Rehabilitation Services Administration sponsored a training program for consumer case manager and human service worker aides (Lefley, 1996). Consumers themselves initiated and ran case management and other service programs, while more client-directed models of case management developed with a focus on building clients' personal strengths (Rapp & Kisthardt, 1996). As the numbers and types of case management continued to proliferate, a leading policy analyst decried, "In concept and in practice, case management appears to be an ill-defined process that lacks substance" (Spitz, 1987, p. 69).

How Many Case Managers? Doubts on the Evaluation Front

By the mid- to late 1980s, state and local mental health authorities were looking for alternate ways to coordinate and oversee service resources. One reason for this was that institutional care was still receiving a large proportion of service funds—nationwide, an average of 70% of mental health expenditures—dollars which were not "following the patient" into the community (Rochefort, 1997; cf. Treffert, 1983). Even where community resources were more developed, dollars were "not following dollars," as local programs absorbed the brunt of inflation rates through constant levels of state appropriations or invested mental health savings in programs other than community care. Medicaid programs were eating into state revenues as well, taking up on average 20% of state budgets and growing at a rate of roughly 10% per year by the late 1980s (Rochefort, 1997). Among the proposals to restructure the financing and provision of care were the establishment of substate authorities charged with coordination of all needed mental health care and supportive services, putting purchasing authority over all state allocations into such an organizational framework, and capitation of funding to providers.

Many of these proposals came together in 1985 in demonstration projects funded by the Robert Wood Johnson (RWJ) Foundation and sponsored by the U.S. Department of Housing and Urban Development. With five years of project funding, nine cities set up centralized local authorities that held clinical, fiscal, and administrative reins over all hospital and community-based mental health services. The authorities controlled pooled funding streams and were expected to provide a full range of services, including those outside of psychiatric care per se, such as social and vocational rehabilitation, housing, and medical and dental care. The centralized accountability, consolidated funding, and comprehensive service system of the RWJ sites typified what would subsequently be known as "public sector managed care" (Hoge, Davidson, Griffith, Sledge, & Howenstine, 1994, p. 1088).

Case management was the main device RWJ sites used to coordinate their comprehensive array of services for individual clients. Indeed, site coordinators saw case management as "the primary intervention introduced or enhanced" through RWJ auspices (Ridgely, Morrissey, Paulson, Goldman, & Calloway, 1996, p. 738). Case managers at these sites had a profile similar to CSP case managers in that they both had graduate-level education and on average seven years experience in mental health care. Also like CSP, they were located in a variety of lead agency offices, including local mental health authorities themselves, specialty case management agencies, and CMHCs. Some case management programs adopted a treatment team model based on the Program for Assertive Community Treatment; more operated on the broker model in which case managers were not clinical care providers.

After several years of the program, a nationwide evaluation of RWJ sites found no consistent evidence of improvement in client outcomes. Research focused on case management suggested that there were still limitations in the availability and adequacy of the community support system that hampered case managers' effectiveness in meeting client needs (Ridgeley et al., 1996). Case managers reported that clients received few services from other community agencies and that, to the extent that clients got psychosocial services (such as training in social skills or health maintenance) or assistance with employment, housing, or entitlements, such service was delivered by the case management program itself. Whether part of treatment teams or not, then, case managers were acting as direct service providers as much as, or more than, service coordinators. In the sites studied, case managers lacked service contacts with over half of the other agencies in the local community support system, especially those outside of mental health care. Moreover, there was no difference in the extent or nature of such contacts between programs using the treatment team approach and those with the broker model, which had been expected to develop a broader service coordination network. Although the amount of case management services clients received increased over the time the program ran, study findings confirmed that "case management by itself did not constitute comprehensive treatment" (Ibid., p. 742).

The RWJ results added to other concerns about case management that had surfaced in mental health program circles in the late 1980s. NIMH had sponsored a carefully controlled study to evaluate how effective and costly case-managed mental health care was compared to those services typically available in a community mental health center (Franklin, Solovitz, Mason, Clemons, & Miller, 1987; Franklin, 1988). People with at least two prior mental hospital stays were randomly assigned to an experimental group to get case management services or a control group, which got other CMHC services but not case management.[11] After 12 months, clients in the case management group showed higher levels of both outpatient and hospital care, with concomitantly higher costs, compared to the control group. There were no major differences between the groups on various measures of psychological well-being and quality of life.

While disappointing to case management proponents, especially within NIMH, these findings did not hamper the spread of such programs. There were, of course, different conclusions that could be drawn other than that case management was ineffective: Perhaps a longer follow-up time was needed; or case management might work best only for some types of clients; or treatment team case management would work better than the broker model; or resource-rich CMHCs could offer adequate services on their own (Franklin et al., 1987; Westermeyer, 1988). A statewide survey in Ohio suggested that case management services might not be providing care as intensive as models assumed: On average, clients got only 13 hours of case management per year, and even clients for whom case management was the main source of service got only about 32 hours per year (Ridgely et al., 1996).

Pending confirmation of these and other possibilities, case management would continue to diffuse through legislative action and administrative fiat, becoming the service most often provided in many local mental health systems. Mental health agencies that did not develop case management components could be at a disadvantage in annual competitions for block grant monies; new program initiatives commonly required case management as a service element. As states continued to struggle with the issues of administering and financing mental health care, case management would emerge at the center of a new organizational strategy, that of managed care.

Managing the Care: Case Management and Managed Behavior Health Care

In the late 1980s and into the 1990s, both private and public sectors looked to managed care to control expenditures for mental health treatment and to rationalize service delivery. It was becoming the norm for health insurance plans to utilize some managed care strategies, whether simply a plan of utilization review or a comprehensive payer/provider institution like an HMO. By 1994, about 82 million individuals had their insurance coverage for mental health and substance abuse treatment covered by some form of managed mental health care program, or, as they were now called, *managed behavioral health care* (MBHC) organizations (Frank & Maguire, 1996). Slightly less than half of these enrollees were members of plans that required services to be received within a network of providers. These plans generally "carved out" their mental health treatment, contracting with specialized, proprietary vendors for management and/or service delivery. The rest of the enrollees were members of more traditional indemnity health insurance plans, in which managed care took the form of "utilization review case management" (Ibid., p. 381) relying on preauthorization and rationing of services on a case-by-case basis. These uses of managed care grew rapidly: By 1996, an estimated 124 million individuals in the private insurance sector had some form of managed mental health care governing their mental health coverage (Rochefort, 1997).

While some individuals with serious mental illness would have received care under these types of arrangements, the services more targeted to that population were still public mental health programs and Medicaid. As states continued to experience fiscal distress into the 1990s, and especially as the promise of more global health care reform proved illusory by mid-decade, the majority of states moved to enroll Medicaid recipients into managed mental health arrangements. These, too, tended to rely on carve-out arrangements separating mental health service provision from that of general health care (Bazeldon Center, 1996; Rochefort, 1997).

Medicaid managed care mental health plans currently encompass a wide array of treatments and services in inpatient, residential, community, and outpatient settings. Case management is a standard feature, although its structure and type vary as much as ever before. While some plans use case management treatment teams like those in the PACT program, more typically case managers are not direct treatment providers. *Utilization review* case management is a relatively new form imported from private managed care. In some plans, this required consumers to call a toll-free number and go through an initial screening with an out-of-state case manager in order to get authorization of services. Controversy over this and other gatekeeping measures within mental health managed care plans has provoked review and new regulations in several states (Rochefort, 1997).

Even where case managers are not the "claims police" (Mullahy, 1996, p. 274), their role in managed care plans has clearly shifted away from that of the hands-on therapeutic agent at the center of CSP. A definition adopted by the developers of the credentialing process for managed care case managers reveals the objectives behind this shift: "Case management is a collaborative process which assesses, plans, implements, coordinates, monitors, and evaluates the options and services required to meet an individual's health needs, using communication and available resources to promote quality, cost-effective outcomes" (Ibid.). The main focus is on promoting a high-quality, cost-effective product. Gone is any hint of advocacy, either at the client or systems level.[12] The envisioned collaboration occurs with all the players and payers involved with the client, including diverse providers and vendors, benefits and insurance claims offices, family members, employers, and others. In many respects, this is a new version of the broker case management role, here coordinating and negotiating among members of a reimbursement network. Like earlier broker case managers, these tend to be paraprofessional workers.

Managed care continues to be controversial, particularly with regard to its implications for client access and choice. Among the concerns about the organization and financing of managed care mental health services are many issues that directly implicate case management. First, limiting clients to a network of providers (however comprehensive) inevitably limits case managers' ability to be client advocates: They cannot easily advocate for care outside the network, and the organizational goals they serve restrict their advocacy within it. Despite the legitimacy these workers may gain by means of a credentialing process, it is difficult to imagine that they have sufficient status to balance out the differences among their collaborators in the ability to control the course, and costs, of care. A second set of issues arises when managed care entities use different providers than those formerly, or concurrently, used by consumers. This then complicates case managers' efforts to provide continuity and coordination. This is particularly likely when clients move between care settings, for example, when discharged from inpatient to outpatient treatment. Few state programs have developed explicit strategies for dealing with such transition issues (Bazeldon Center, 1996). At the systems level, because managed care carries with it financial risk, it can exacerbate problems of cost- and care-shifting between Medicaid and public mental health systems, as organizations try to avoid responsibility for the most severely ill (Frank & Maguire, 1996). Case managers may be caught in the middle here, having to execute decisions about which clients not to serve or to pull together a care package with additional bureaucratic layers.

Two Decades of Case Management: The Product and Agent of Public Policy

Surveying the array of approaches that followed the CSP initiative, one commentary likened case management to a "Rorschach test" onto which "an individual, an agency, or a community will project . . . its own particular solution to the problems it faces in providing community-based care for the chronic mentally ill" (Schwartz, Goldman, & Churgin, 1982, p. 1006). Close to two decades later, the same can be said for case management as an instrument of public policy. Its initial goals of increasing access and coordinating services transformed with the policy climate to those of service efficiency and cost-effectiveness.

Throughout this time, case management has been a practice with diverse forms and missions and of variable and questionable effectiveness. Contradictions in this practice abound: "charged with overcoming environmental barriers for clients . . . [case managers] have in fact little power or authority to do so" (Ellison, Rogers, Sciarappa, Cohen, & Forbess, 1995, p. 111). Faced with inadequate community resources, case managers often become direct service providers. In communities richer in programs, case management becomes redundant, itself a duplicated service. As cost constraint becomes a paramount policy focus, the ability of case managers to be client advocates—always a precarious and underdeveloped attribute of their role—appears to dissolve: "Although case managers are expected to have close interpersonal contact with clients and to intercede and advocate on their behalf, in fact, case management is a product and an agent of the public policy that funds it" (Ibid.).

The contradictions of case management practice reflect broader incongruities embedded in the policies, ideologies, and ethos that drove the practice's development. Primary among these was the belief that the problems encountered with deinstitutionalization could be solved through a more effective and rational organization of services. Notwithstanding the diversity of its goals and structures, case management is always an instrument of service rationalization; that is, an attempt to organize service systems more effectively. The implicit faith accorded this approach by key actors within NIMH, state systems, and the mental health professions provided both rationale and grounding for CSP, and it is doubtful that case management would have achieved such prominence in the mental health sector absent this broader ethos of rationalization. What this stance ignored, however, were the broader structural sources of service fragmentation: the turf interests of providers in different sectors and of governmental bureaucracies, particularly at the state level; or the ideological as well as resource gulf between welfare-linked programs (such as SSI and Medicaid) and those with universal entitlements (such as CMHCs). Although later programs (such as the RWJ initiatives and early managed care arrangements) attempted more ambitious forms of rationalization that created new structures of care, they still relied on case managers to overcome service fragmentation on a case-by-case basis.

A second element underlying the pervasive development of case management was the search for ways to maintain, or even expand, the availability of publicly funded services without inflating public costs. This quest lay behind the rise of the "contracting regime" (Smith & Lipsky, 1993, p. 43) and the creation of paraprofessional positions. Both trends augmented support for case management as a policy tool, making for unlikely alliances among public, nonprofit, and proprietary service agencies, or between mental health professionals and the unions representing paraprofessional workers. That it might be fundamentally incongruent to try to maintain service levels while controlling costs became apparent with the hardening of states' economies in the 1980s; this did not, however, fail to derail case management's momentum. For one reason, case management offered contracting agencies several advantages: It connected them with funding streams, especially once mandated as part of state programs; and it was adaptable to different styles of service provision, requiring little in the way of change by service agencies in order to provide it. The continued contradiction between service expansion and cost restraint would fall on the shoulders of the case managers themselves, requiring them to balance roles as gatekeepers, service advocates, and direct providers of care that was otherwise unavailable.

Yet, there were also other logics at work in the use of case management to put a human face on increasingly distant service bureaucracies. The notion of a case manager as a "traveling companion" (Deitchman, 1980, p. 789) reflects a realization of the pervasive and long-term consequences of chronic mental illness. The dovetailing of case management with the mental health advocacy and consumer movements, through peer case managers and consumer-run programs, built on the recognition that to be good traveling companions case managers needed empathy and a personal relationship with their clients. The ethic of care underlying these aspects of case management centers on flexible and individualized understandings of client problems and possible solutions, rather than standardized, rationalized approaches. It values client perspectives over clinical or bureaucratic abstractions and aims at personal development (or, in clinical terms, "psychosocial rehabilitation") rather than cost-effectiveness (McAuley, Teaster, & Safewright, 1999).

Case management in mental health thus developed with two equally prominent faces: that of the system rationalizer, a formal organizational role; and that of a caring, personal connection, more like a member of a family or other "primary group" (Dill, 1987). Based on different aims and types of social relations, these two orientations build into the role of case manager diverse and often contradictory expectations. The final section examines the implications of this for case management practice today.

MENTAL HEALTH CASE MANAGEMENT IN PRACTICE

Case managers are now part of every type of service program providing mental health care: community mental health centers; mental health carveouts in managed care plans; discharge planning in psychiatric hospitals; consumer-directed programs; mental health associations; substance abuse treatment facilities; and the myriad other community treatment facilities. A central element in services for clients with chronic disorders, case management is a mandate of CSS service provision in most states. Given the deep-seated contradictions in case management's past, as well as the variety of programs offering it at present, it is not surprising that there is little consistency in the structure and form of case management, and little clarity or coherence in its practice. The following outlines in broad strokes who case managers are and how they work, highlighting the sources of diversity among them.

A Snapshot View

As was true from its inception, case management continues to provide a relatively low-level professional position, especially when viewed in the context of the professional mental health hierarchy (Cnaan, 1994; Ellison et al., 1995; Hromco, Lyons, & Nikkel, 1997). In one recent national survey of case managers serving persons with severe psychiatric disability, case managers tended to be young, female, trained at the bachelor's level, and professionally identified with social work (Ellison et al., 1995). Substantial numbers had less education and no professional self-identification. Their supervisors, in contrast, were more likely to be older, male, and educated at the master's level, and less identified with social work. Programs and states vary considerably in the characteristics of case managers, however; for example, a survey across three states found 60% of Oregon's CMHC case managers trained at the master's level, compared to 12.1% in Indiana and 15.3% in Illinois (Hromco et al., 1997).

As seen historically, several varieties or models of case management have evolved, at times in connection with specific programmatic approaches. Models prominently featured in the program evaluation literature include the broker or generalist model, clinical case management, the intensive case management (ICM) model, the Assertive Community Treatment (ACT) team model, the Personal Strengths model, and the rehabilitation model.[13] These models differ along many dimensions, including caseload features, range and types of services, focus of objectives, locus of contacts, target population, and extent and form of client involvement and control (Mueser, Bond, Drake, & Resnick, 1998; Rapp & Kisthardt, 1996; Pescosolido et al., 1995). In practice, however, there appears to be great overlap among different models in the structure and functions of associated programs (Huxley & Warner, 1992; Rapp, 1998), leading the reviewers of a decade of outcome literature to conclude, "It is difficult if not impossible to ascertain similarities and differences between interventions with other than broad strokes" (Chamberlain and Rapp, 1991, p. 174). Moreover, few programs appear to identify in terms of an ideal model; for example, one national survey of case managers found less than one-fourth describing their program as following a definite model, with the Personal Strengths model having the greatest representation at 12% (Ellison et al., 1995). Meta-analyses of evaluation research have demonstrated that different case management models do not differ clearly or significantly in terms of program effectiveness (Gorey et al., 1998; Mueser et al., 1998).[14] Case management models thus seem to be more differentiated as ideal types, than in practice.

There is also little consistency among case management programs in terms of basic elements of practice. Different surveys have found case-loads, for example, averaging 25 to 30 clients per case manager, but with ranges of from 1:1 to 1:300 (Ellison et al., 1995; Hromco, Lyons, & Nikkel, 1995; cf. Mueser et al., 1998). Programs' missions and values are even more variable: Beyond a general dedication to preventing hospitalization, a nationwide sample of case managers found no other mission ranked high in importance by the majority of respondents (Ellison et al., 1995). Very few ranked as important clinical goals such as reducing symptoms.[15] Case managers in this study also showed no coherent set of values governing their practice: While values reflecting a focus on client's well-being and rights (such as individualization, normalization, empowerment, and dignity) ranked first among the values programs tried to uphold, none of these values was ranked first by more than 15% of respondents. Moreover, there was no overall correlation among the values, missions, and activities of the programs.

Greater clarity emerges from descriptions of case managers' activities in this survey, since almost all reported doing client assessments of different types. The most common formal assessment was, however, a clinical standard, namely, the mental status exam; and substantial proportions of case managers did not report assessing clients' level of functioning, interests, or skills. Beyond assessment, there was less consistency either in the extent to which case managers report doing other activities, or in their rating of activities as important. Only "linking clients to service providers" and "intervening during client crises" received high ranking by the majority of case managers in this study; furthermore, case managers did not consistently report doing advocacy, relationship-building, formal skill training, or "monitoring," nor did the majority rank those as important in their repertoire. Other researchers confirm that case managers' time is dominated by work that is not client-centered, especially administrative tasks and paperwork (Hromco et al., 1997; Hamner & Bryant, 1997; Cnaan, 1994).

That activities usually considered core case management functions appear peripheral while the main focus is on such tasks as assessment and crisis intervention indicates that case management practice is still largely "system-driven": "Case managers primarily focus on compensating for fragmented, uncoordinated services, which leave clients open to crises, rather than on 'client-driven' elucidation of needs and desired interventions" (Ellison et al., 1995, p. 110). This is particularly true in areas with fewer or less accessible services, where programs adapt to system inadequacies through increased caseloads, conducting little advocacy or service development, and limiting responses primarily to clients most in need (Clark, Landis, & Fisher, 1990).

What case management is, then, may depend on what case managers can do: In service-poor environments, case managers can be stuck in a crisis-response mode filling in directly for missing service pieces (Ibid.; cf. Fisher, Landis, & Clark, 1988). In communities with more resources, case management programs run the risk of themselves being redundant (cf. Solomon et al., 1986), but may also develop more elaborate roles including skill training and direct therapy (Hromco et al., 1995). Not surprisingly, assessments of the predictors of the amount of service time case managers provide suggest that client characteristics are less important than factors related to the overall level and duration of care (Hamner & Bryant, 1997; Clark et al., 1990).

"The Party's in Here": Contradictions in Case Management Practice

Mental health case managers occupy complex roles. On the one hand, they are responsible for connecting clients with the service system and thus perform in much the same people-processing mode characteristic of case managers in long-term care. As we saw in Chapter 2, this requires them to work as a boundary spanner, connecting their program with other service agencies and responding to a multitude of organizational needs and objectives. But for mental health care, case managers are also directly involved in trying to change clients, that is, to affect clients' behavior, cognition, or emotional well-being. They do this by being therapists themselves, by working as part of clinical teams, and/or by taking on clinical activities. As "people-changers," they are trying to induce fundamental alterations in clients' social roles, helping clients develop the skills and behavior needed to be successful community residents. Doing this requires long-term contact with clients and the socialization that comes with a personal, as well as professional, relationship (cf. Hasenfeld, 1972). Case managers must thus balance their responsibilities within the service delivery system with the demands of their relationships with clients. In what follows, we examine some of the contradictions that emerge from this, illustrating them with material drawn from a study of individuals with chronic mental illness residing in a midsize Northeastern city.[16]

As they attempt to help clients maintain stable residence in the community, case managers encounter the very limitations in services that make community living difficult. What they offer clients can thus fall short because of systems' gaps, and enabling clients to choose among inadequate services cannot be "empowering." This is clear in the case of "Al," a man in his early thirties who had been diagnosed with schizophrenia over a decade before. Following several hospitalizations and a stay in a group home, Al now lives alone in a small apartment, supported by SSI. The low level of support this provides is stressful for Al, and he would like to find a job. He knows that his inconsistent job history works against him; he had left one job without giving notice and was fired from his last job for getting involved in a fight. Still, he is disappointed in the efforts of programs designed to help mental health consumers get jobs and has not found other mental health services useful, either. From the perspective of the service system, Al could easily be seen as a difficult and "treatment-resistant" client. From Al's perspective, the system offered him nothing of meaning:

The employment service? Well, they didn't have . . . any links, they didn't have any connections, like, I thought I could just go to their office and, you know, apply for jobs that I would get . . . but there were jobs, well best one they could offer was like mopping the floor at a store, or . . . they wanted me to work at Wendy's and stuff like that, I just wouldn't do it . . . I'd love to have a job. I figured they'd just ease me into some place you know, [but] they don't know anybody there, or, you know you have to have a degree, or, it's a million miles away, you don't have a car. So, we got frustrated and, uh, thought it was kind of futile after a while, just thought I'd had enough, if you're not going to get anything good for me . . . I don't need the services.

The lack of meaningful opportunities for productive and social activity robs many people with chronic mental illness of the sense of being a valued member of society. Restricted social networks and loneliness are also perpetual problems for many of these individuals (Osgood, 1992; Dozier & Franklin, 1988; Goering et al., 1992). Psychiatric conditions and low tolerance for stress contribute to this isolation and social disability, but the system of mental health services creates its own form of isolation, illustrated in the following hypothetical case:

Roger lives with three other mental health clients in a duplex in a nice neighborhood. Agency staff help him with daily living tasks and collect his rent. Once a month with the help of their case manager, Roger, his housemates, and the four clients living in the next duplex get together for an enjoyable dinner and a video. Three days a week Roger goes to a rehabilitation program to learn work skills. In the afternoons he hangs out at an agency drop-in center, sometimes going to their special "double trouble" group for persons with mental illness and alcohol problems. On evenings and weekends, Roger usually watches TV, drinks a few beers, and cares for his aquarium of tropical fish. His favorite person is Chris, a support worker who shares his interest in fish. Sometimes they go look at fish in a pet store. (Curtis, 1994, p. 1)

While "Roger" may seem to be living successfully on an independent basis, it is clearly a bracketed independence. Roger's connections with work, recreation, transportation, and other provisions of everyday life reflect a community support system that is relatively well endowed and co-ordinated, no doubt through the efforts of case managers. To the extent that he has integrated into a community, however, it is a community of service providers and other consumers. This is particularly likely to happen for people in supported housing situations, for whom paid staff and coresidents can replace family and other friends, becoming the major part of personal networks (Goering et al., 1992; cf. Rowe, 1999). Attempts to rationalize and coordinate service systems may thus have the unintended and ironic consequence of re-creating the mental institution without walls, an island of support cut off from the mainland of society.

What is problematic for case managers here is to provide support without creating dependency; and to nurture hope even when clients may never leave the system of care. This is evident from this study in the case of a couple, George and Frances, both of whom are mental health consumers. George got Barbara as a case manager through the public mental health agency roughly three years before the interview. Barbara describes her role as being "the overseer of . . . services" for George, making sure that he gets the care he needs. She sees him at least once a month as part of monitoring his service plan; she also makes occasional informal visits. Although assigned only to George, Barbara acknowledges the needs of the two as a couple and includes Frances in discussions, as well as takes them out together to receive a service or just to talk. In addition to Barbara, George and Frances receive ongoing care through a program offering support for community living, which has connected them with a social worker and a volunteer who provides transportation and social activities. Apart from Frances' family, the couple's social network appears to consist almost entirely of Barbara, the social worker, the volunteer, and other participants in the community living program. Neither George nor Frances is employed: George, who describes himself as having schizophrenia, has held a series of jobs for very short times since his release from a prolonged stay in a psychiatric hospital; Frances has never been employed other than briefly in a sheltered workshop.

Insight into the nature of the couple's relationship with the case manager emerged when, during the interview, Barbara made an unscheduled visit. Expecting that their social worker would also arrive shortly to take Frances to her first visit to a new therapist, Frances joked, "The party's in here. . . . Put a sign on the door, the party is in here." In the midst of the interview, Barbara noted that she had helped George take on some small jobs: "Another of my clients [moved] into another apartment; and it was kinda like, stopping by like now, and 'gee are you interested [in helping move the client],' because I was able to give him $20 for helping out, and he was grateful." Agreeing with the interviewer's remark that George was a good worker, Barbara added, "He stays really focused. Uh, he didn't have to be told what to do; and yet he . . . was comfortable for the other people to be around. And I think for him to commit himself to having to do this all the time would be difficult, but he is able to, you know, short-term."

Barbara appears here to be attempting to set realistic goals for George, negotiating between his expectations and those of others in society. This aspect of her role was further evident when shortly thereafter Barbara responded to critical remarks offered by George, and more particularly by Frances, indicating that George's psychiatrist unreasonably expects George to find work: "She's, she's not putting pressure on you [George]. She does bring up the subject but she's, she's not being real rigid about it." George responds, "Uh-huh. Uh. Uh. No." The conversation continued:

> Barbara: She thinks that maybe you need more organization to your day. And that you might feel better about that. But, she's not . . . she promotes this, and she reminds them that they can continue to set higher goals. You know, but she doesn't push them to the point that that's going to be un-comfortable, you know. So. Although with [George], that's kind of stuck in his head, because she does mention it. "Well, what have you been do-ing? Have you been looking for a job?"
> Frances: Yea, but she shouldn't pressure you like that.
> Barbara: Oh, she's not.
> George: No.

Barbara has done what she can here to make a smoother connection to the professional service system. Neither Frances nor George appears con-vinced, however, and their response to the psychiatrist appears to be as much related to the lack of good options for George as to the psychiatrist's goals: As Frances exclaims, "Hey, what does she expect you to do? A hop, skip, and a jump to find work."

While Barbara sees her role as making service connections for George and keep them running smoothly, she encounters multiple barriers in per-forming that role. Toward the end of her visit, she asks whether George and Frances will be attending a party at the community living program. Frances replies that they would like to go, but they have no ride since their volunteer won't be going. Both Barbara and the social worker explain that they have already committed to giving other people rides. After several rounds about the issue, Barbara tells Frances, "I'll call if I come up with anything, [but]. . . . If you don't hear from me . . ." It appears that the only party George and Frances will have attended that week will be the one in their own apartment. While on the surface a trivial incident, it is telling that without their service providers' assistance George and Frances are de-prived of social activity. While Barbara might like to promote George's in-dependent functioning to the extent his condition allows, she does so in the context of a relationship in which he is inevitably at least partially dependent.

The nature of this relationship—a personal connection and trust, built up over time—may, however, be the most important aspect of case management practice. Studies show that clients value the quality of their bonds with case managers, and that their perceptions of that relationship are related to, and may even predict, the success of community care programs (see reviews in Mueser et al., 1998, and Rapp, 1998). Indeed, low-key, face-to-face contacts—the building blocks of the connection—may be more conducive to client well-being than formal service connections (Huxley & Warner, 1992). It is not always clear, however, what the appropriate boundaries and content of the relationship are, nor how to address the conflicts that case managers inherit from the multiple aspects of their role (cf. Rowe, 1999).

The consumer movement offers an alternative approach to mental health care based on the advantages of connecting with a peer, such as empathy, role modeling, and knowledge of concrete survival skills (Lefley, 1996; Trainor, Shepherd, Boydell, Leff, & Crawford, 1997). While some consumer programs provide peer case management directly, most perform various case management functions such as informing consumers of available services; providing ongoing social contact, support, and coaching; or offering crisis intervention through hot line telephone programs. But the focus is deliberately different from that of professional services, with the emphasis on consumers playing a central role in choosing, controlling, and coordinating the services they receive (Trainor et al., 1997; Deegan, 1992; see also the discussion of peer modeling forms of case management in Albrecht & Peters, 1997).

"Kathy," the person in this community care study who was most involved with consumer-directed mental health initiatives, actively case managed her own care, seeking out closer relationships with service providers with whom she felt a more personal connection. This did not include her present case manager, with whom Kathy disagreed about her service needs and whom she bypassed in at least one attempt to get care. At the time of our interview, Kathy's closest connection was with a social worker who shared one of her diagnoses; commenting on her own ambition to go into social work, Kathy noted, "[The social worker] is a great social worker, because she's been through it. You know, she can talk to me on a personal level, and . . . that's sort of like a role model for me."

Consumer-directed programs attempt to foster just this type of role modeling, using it to leverage the consumer out of the client role and into one of self-direction. Studies of consumer groups in a major provincial initiative in Canada found members reporting significant impacts of the program on their self-confidence and sense of being in control and able to cope (Trainor et al., 1997). Contrary to concerns that involvement in consumer-only groups might lock members in a mental health ghetto, this research found that members increased their social contacts in the wider community, with consumers and nonconsumers as well, while decreasing their use of formal mental health services. Ranking the helpfulness and/or harmfulness of various organizations and providers, members ranked other consumers and themselves as the most helpful, higher than any category of mental health professional. In contrast, they ranked case managers ninth (of 12 categories), with a rating close to the midpoint between "helpful" and "harmful." Many of the ways members said consumer groups helped them fell within the traditional rubric of case management, such as providing knowledge about available services and resources.

More generally, the consumer movement appears to concentrate on the advocacy role case management has so often abjured. In some cases, consumer programs directly engage in economic activities, policy development, and mutual support. Overall, the philosophy of mutual aid and self-help within the movement emphasizes "justice for psychiatric consumers/survivors as individuals and as a class" (*In Profile*, 1994). Assessing consumer initiatives in her state, Kathy pointed to the necessity of this dual-level advocacy: "I mean, [the state] talks about consumer empowerment and all, . . . it's something that they're really into . . . but when it comes down to the bucks, we have no say. . . . I'd like consumers to have the power to . . . say where some money goes. You know, right now it depends on the big administrators."

Consumer programs take different tacks in attempting to gain this fiscal and administrative control. Some consumer advocates favor the development of personal care attendants managed by the consumer (similar to those developed by the independent living movement for people with disabilities) as a substitute for services secured by a professional case manager (Fischer, 1994). Other programs have provided consumers with vouchers they can use to purchase community support goods and services or pool to fund new programs (Bertsch, 1992). While giving consumers more control over service dollars, these programs still rely on case managers and other providers to monitor the voucher process.

Within the context of the whole mental health system, consumers are still cast primarily in the role of "adjunct"; that is, as "advisors, planners, and in some cases, as staff members" (Trainor et al., 1997, p. 138) of services. Consumer direction based on a more global model of mutual aid and self-help remains a vision enacted in alternative programs (cf. Carling, 1995), while the overall structure of the service system remains intact, and with it the conditions still promoting, and complicating, case management.

CONCLUSION: LOOKING TO THE FUTURE

The dilemmas of case management practice highlight more fundamental dilemmas of our mental health care system. Case management programs are, and have always been, aimed as much at the needs of that system and its service providers as at those of clients: needs for stable funding, employment of workers, cost containment, rationalized production, and coordinated service provision. Contradictions abound not only among those aims, but also between them and objectives of providing high-quality, accessible care. Case management's success within the system owes much to its use as part of larger battles and contested domains arising from those contradictions. Yet the contending demands on mental health care leave case managers caught in the middle: "In effect, case managers are being asked—individually and repeatedly—to resolve the conflicts between competing claims on health care resources that agencies, programs, and society at large have not yet been able to resolve, and with few guidelines and little support" (Padgett, 1998, pp. 5–6).

The lack of clear definition of key aspects of case management—what it is; what it does; whether it is effective, and for whom—has not dampened its entrenchment within the system. Indeed, case management has come to seem a normal, even natural, part of any attempt to provide comprehensive mental health services. This should not be surprising, given that other critical aspects of mental health care, such as its quality, are equally resistant to clarity. Moreover, the main trends in mental health policy—including privatization, cost containment, and service rationalization—have emerged based on dominant assumptions about the desirable properties of the system. Programs taking these as a given share in the "moral weight" (Ibid.) of the trend at large, whether or not their contribution to particular objectives can be documented.

The programmatic success of case management has come, however, at some expense to the case manager's role as a client's agent. The boundaries of that role have always been set within a framework of the care available within the system, or provided through case managers' own auspices. Pharmaceutical advances and new types of service structures have expanded that framework; countervailing forces of cost restraint, supply management, and public sector retrenchment have contracted it. Seen in this context, providing and coordinating care are not the matters of individual options and choice envisioned by the rubric of case management. It is doubtful that any one program can balance the best interests of mental health providers, insurers, consumers, family members, and the state; yet this is still the expectation for case managers.

Close to 40 years after deinstitutionalization, mental health care appears to be building momentum and poised for significant advances. Mental health advocates at state and federal levels are pushing for parity in insurance coverage between mental and physical health care. Community programs, presidential candidates, and the Surgeon General proclaim the need to end the stigma attached to mental illness. State mental health systems are directing service dollars toward programs increasing the employment of people with chronic mental illness. Yet parity will not go far enough if millions of Americans (an estimated 45 million at this writing) remain without health insurance. Antistigma programs cannot fully succeed as long as people with chronic psychiatric disability must depend on social welfare systems for their health care and livelihood. As seen in the next chapter, jobs programs cannot serve everyone, nor do they alone provide the foundation for meeting clients' basic needs.

Case management will continue to be a main way we attempt to compensate for the shortcomings of our service system. A danger with the new proposals is that they may add more interests to be balanced and place more moral claims on the system in general and the case manager's role in particular. To the extent that reimbursement structures provide more incentive to assign case managers to vocational programs, for example, case managers will absorb the claims of the work ethic and the interests of potential employers. If, in the process, socialization programs become a residual placement for case managers, their aims will likewise become secondary.[17] On a broader level, if parity efforts succeed, they will almost certainly be accompanied by greater attempts to control the supply and costs of both physical and mental health care. Those efforts will most likely be funneled through the actions of case managers, further distancing them from their role as client agents, advocates, or traveling companions.

For these to be acceptable trade-offs, there must be both better knowledge and explicit approval of their consequences. Case management programs have proven adaptable to diverse policy climates and objectives; they will have no difficulty adjusting to any foreseeable programmatic demands. While others—from consumer peers and family members to legal advocates and ombudspeople—can and do travel beside those with chronic mental illness, no one spans the borders of the formal and informal institutions comprising the mental health system as deliberately as case managers. For case managers to lose the basis for their personal connection with clients will only increase the latter's vulnerability and that of our system of mental health care as a whole.

NOTES

1. The definition of mental illness has long been subject to contention and revision (Mechanic, 1980; Rochefort, 1989). At the most general level, "severe and chronic mental illness" refers to a heterogeneous category including schizophrenia, major mood disorders, and other psychotic and organic illnesses. *Severe* denotes the occurrence of episodic symptoms with dysfunctional consequences; *chronic,* that the condition is persistent and long-term. For the purposes of this chapter, the relevant meanings are those formulated within the policies and programs in which case management devel-

oped. The 1980 National Plan for the Chronically Mentally Ill formulated by a steering committee of the Department of Health and Human Services offered a comprehensive definition that reads in part:

> The chronically mentally ill population encompasses persons who suffer certain mental or emotional disorders (organic brain syndrome, schizophrenia, recurrent depressive and manic-depressive disorders, paranoid and other psychoses, plus other disorders that may become chronic) that erode or prevent the development of their functional capacities in relation to (three or more of) such primary aspects of daily life as personal hygiene and self-care, self-direction, inter-personal relationships, social transactions, learning, and recreation, and that erode or prevent the development of their economic self-sufficiency . . . (Department of Health and Human Services, 1981, p. 2–11)

The definition goes on to discuss the nature of institutional and other treatment received by such individuals and their risk for repeated hospitalization. Notable here is the emphasis on functioning, economic self-sufficiency, and institutionalization as attributes of the individuals in a category otherwise denoted by psychiatric diagnosis and chronic disorder. Together, these attributes underscore the importance of adequate support in community settings, the core of the emerging "national plan," a key element of which was case management.

2. For a comprehensive history of deinstitutionalization and mental health policy, see Grob (1991). Other systematic analyses are to be found in Aviram, Syme, and Cohen (1976), Bell (1989), Brown (1985), Grob (1994), Gronfein (1985), Mechanic (1980), Rochefort (1997), Rose (1979), and Scull (1976).

3. With reference to the Community Mental Health Centers Act of 1963, for example, a basic division occurs between a view highlighting the "progressive" role of activist reformers, federal officials, and Congress members (Foley, 1975) versus those adopting political economic perspectives that see the act in the context of psychiatric expansionism extending social control to community-based care (Scull, 1976; Brown, 1985; see discussion in Rochefort [1997]).

4. Concerns about the homeless mentally ill would mount over the next decade, as the growing ranks of homeless people drew social attention and outrage. An American Psychiatric Association Task Force would conclude that homelessness among the chronic mentally ill was caused by the failures of community resources to replace the total responsibility for patient care the mental hospital had assumed—including the coordination of basic physical and social needs. At the same time, claiming that some seriously ill people would always have need for the sanctuary of the hospital, the task force recommended legal changes to facilitate involuntary civil commitment (Lamb & Talbott, 1986; cf. LaFond & Durham, 1992).

5. See Platman et al. (1982) and Turner and TenHoor (1978) for detailed accounts of the history of CSP.

6. The connection was completely intentional. Early NIMH task forces used drafts of BSS literature in forming ideas for the CSP, and later circulated

their drafts to BSS developers for feedback. See Turner and TenHoor (1978).

7. Deitchman (National Institute of Mental Health, 1982, p. 118), for example, notes charges that case mangers are "just 'mental health hucksters' who have redefined what they've always done to fit new Federal guidelines, to get new Federal dollars."

8. Rochefort (1993) provides a detailed review of the consequences of the ADAMH block grant for CMHCs, noting that the effects were as much administrative and political and fiscal. ADAMH placed CMHCs much more under state authority than they had been formerly, and one reason for their fate may have been their "'historically . . . adversarial relation with state mental health departments'" (p. 81).

9. Some people did not receive Medicaid due to restrictive SSI criteria, although these were successfully challenged in court actions later in the 1980s (Rochefort, 1997). Others received secondary insurance under Medicare, which disqualified them from PCCM (Bazeldon Center for Mental Health Law, 1996).

10. Detroit, for example, experienced a 32% increase in the caseloads of chronically mentally ill clients of primary mental health agencies from 1981 to 1983, while its budget for mental health programs increased 4% in constant dollars over that period (Burt & Pittman, 1985, pp. 96–97).

11. The case management was of the generalist or broker type, with case managers not providing clinical services.

12. The author later refers to case managers as "impartial advocates" (Mullahy, 1996, p. 274), at best a serious dilution of the original advocacy role of case management and at worst an oxymoron.

13. For descriptions, comparisons, and evaluations of these approaches, as well as overviews of pertinent literature on each, see Pescosolido et al., 1995; Rapp and Kisthardt, 1996; Chamberlain and Rapp, 1991; Solomon, 1992; Schmidt-Posner and Jerrell, 1998; Mueser et al., 1998; Rapp, 1998; and Gorey et al., 1998.

14. Comparisons are beset by the same methodological problems that abound in evaluating the efficacy of all case management programs. Surveying the evidence for case management in this area leads one analyst to conclude

> Do the foregoing studies justify current claims that case management has been shown to be effective with seriously mentally ill individuals? These studies' mixed results and the uneven quality of their research designs leaves plenty of room for cognitive dissonance factors to influence different reviewers to draw different conclusions. In this reviewer's interpretation, the answer is no. The inconsistent results fall short of providing conclusive evidence that any case management models are effective . . . neither do they offer conclusive evidence that case management is ineffective. (Rubin, 1992, pp. 144–145)

There nonetheless appears to be consensus that the brokerage model in which case managers act primarily as referral agents is not as effective as other approaches in which there is more intensive and/or clinical involvement (see Mueser et al., 1998; and Rapp & Kisthardt, 1996). The efficacy of the ACT approach is well supported in the literature (see review in Mueser et al., 1998), but it is unclear what or how much is contributed by particular case management features. Other research reviews suggest that all case management clients on average do better than those not receiving such intervention, that caseload size is the only feature of case management programs clearly (and negatively) related to client outcomes (Gorey et al., 1998), and that case management programs (with the exception of brokers) tend to achieve their primary objectives regardless of the particular focus of the intervention (Chamberlain and Rapp, 1991). For discussion of practice guidelines emerging from an overall comparison of case management models, see Rapp (1998).

15. These perceptions find expression as well in the outcomes of case management programs. As Solomon (1992, p. 177) notes, "Case management is a system management service more so than a clinical service. . . . Therefore, it is not surprising that case management appears to affect system outcomes, e.g., rehospitalization, more than clinical outcomes."

16. The Springfield Study of Populations with Disabilities (Susan M. Allen, P.I.), supported in part by grant no. 19678 from the Robert Wood Johnson Foundation. Case material comes from the qualitative component of this study, for which the author trained fieldworkers conducting in-depth interviews with 50 respondents with a range of disabilities, including 10 with diagnoses of persistent mental illness. See Allen and Mor (1997, 1998) for a description of the study and its broader findings.

17. As noted by F. L. Paranzino, ACSW, Newport County Community Mental Health Center, in personal communication, Middletown, R.I., November 18, 1999.

4

"Not Alms But a Friend"

Case Management and Social Welfare

Despite the optimism of the above motto,[1] adopted by the Boston Associated Charities in 1879, a wide gulf separates the social work ideal of case management as the "friendly face" of an impersonal bureaucracy and the reality of case management practice in public welfare.[2] Indeed, many within the social service sector consider *welfare case management* an oxymoron, its actuality precluded by incompatible objectives and intentionally scarce resources. Yet welfare programs have relied on case managers for over two decades, and the success of current welfare reform hinges on their effectiveness. This chapter explores the sources of these contradictions and their consequences for welfare workers and recipients.

Despite their recency, case management programs here have an institutional history outstripping that of any service arena save other fields of welfare. They are grounded in the casework approach of social work, which evolved as part of private charities' attempts to redress the problems occasioned by industrialization and immigration in the late 19th century. The federal program most associated with public welfare, Aid to Families with Dependent Children (AFDC), initially centered on the provision of social services and social casework, anticipating both the rationale and the functions of case management projects. Through the late 1960s and 1970s the concept of service integration guided the development of antipoverty programs, child welfare services, and experiments in community development, and with these came case management practice. As federal commitments retrenched from the 1970s onward, the main route for expansion of public welfare services became contracts with the private sector, resulting in a complicated network of funding and service relationships. Within this context the first case-managed welfare-to-work projects arose as state-level demonstration efforts, culminating in 1988 with the embodiment of case management as an optional service within the federally sponsored Job Opportunities and Basic Skills (JOBS) program.

This chapter highlights the impact of three related forces in the history of social welfare forging the development of case management. The first derives from the fragmentation of welfare provision created by divisions within and among public and private sectors. The product of a "reluctant welfare state," this decentralized system in turn fragmented services at the client level and led to the creation of corporatist alliances between public and private agencies. Both of these situations encouraged case management strategies.

The second force consists of social images and moral constructions attached to the provision and the recipients of public aid. While the history of American welfare reveals the interplay of differing, often contradictory perceptions and moral constructs, principles of "deservingness," dependency, and the work ethic have formed a core fashioned to the needs of particular times. Linked to the gender, racial, and class divisions of American society, these principles have shaped welfare policy by fueling political rhetoric and public support for programs aiding only those deemed worthy, and then only for as long as they could not support themselves. The principles also underlie the goals and focus of welfare-to-work case management. More generally, negative images surrounding both the recipient and the provider of welfare increase the conflict and friction already inherent in case management practice.

The third force leading social welfare to case management channeled through the profession of social work, which has claimed welfare as its domain much as medicine has claimed health care. At key junctions, social work leaders have sought to control the direction of social welfare in ways advancing the perspective and status of the profession. Professional associations promoted first social casework and, later, case management as technological advances that would help achieve welfare policy goals. In the process, they embedded professional roles in a highly bureaucratized setting, an uneasy combination that continues to affect case management practice.

These forces are intertwined threads running through the history of social welfare policy in the United States. To demonstrate this, we first track each separately across critical eras in the development of the American welfare state from the Progressive era through the 1970s. We then see the three twined together in the conservative revolution from the 1980s onward, transforming the goal of public policy first to "welfare-to-work," and then to "ending welfare as we know it." Case management provides a vehicle for these shifts, and we will examine the origins and role of case management within the JOBS program, the federal initiative bridging the policy changes of the last decade. Finally, we see how these forces are still evident in case management practices, and especially in relations between welfare providers and recipients.

SOCIAL WELFARE POLICY AND THE
COURSES OF CASE MANAGEMENT

The Reluctant Welfare State

Like long-term care and mental health services, public welfare programs comprise a decentralized mixture of private efforts with public ones at federal, state, and local levels. Direct services are provided less by public auspices than through them, in complicated contractual arrangements. While in this broad framework the welfare sector differs little from the others of interest, it is the product of forces distinct both in degree and in kind. In particular, welfare today bears the legacy of an aversion to acknowledging its functions as a global public responsibility.

The limited federal role in assuring minimal standards of basic goods such as income, nutrition, health, and housing evoked the label "reluctant welfare state" from Harold Wilensky and Charles Lebeaux in a classic treatise on social policy in the mid-1960s (Wilensky & Lebeaux, 1965). Those authors deemed the American reliance on state, local, and voluntary means of social protection regressive relative to the commitments of governments in other industrialized countries. At its core, our welfare policy has been hesitant to extend social protection as a matter of citizen entitlement; this translates programmatically into means-tested, targeted programs perennially subject to reform and retraction (Smith & Lipsky, 1993).

Among welfare programs, none has been more emblematic of the reluctant state than income maintenance, known historically as *public relief*. Modeled on the English Poor Law, relief had been the purview of local and religious authorities from colonial times until the latter half of the 19th century. President Franklin Pierce, in vetoing a bill in 1854 to provide public land for the building of special hospitals for the insane, blind, and deaf, reinforced the responsibility of the states in this arena: "I can not find any authority in the Constitution for making the Federal Government the great almoner of public charity. . . . And if it were admissible . . . I can not avoid the belief that it would in the end be prejudicial . . . to the noble offices of charity" (cited in Axinn & Levin, 1997, p. 47). As economic dislocations caused by the Civil War, immigration, urbanization, and industrialization submerged meager local and state capacities, private charities and mutual aid societies arose in great numbers. Their leaders formed Charity Organization Societies (COSs) to synchronize their activities for several purposes: to expedite service delivery, to eliminate duplication of services, and to deter public control (Kagan & Neville, 1993). Soon active in all major cities, COSs would dominate the provision of social welfare services throughout the last quarter of the 19th century. Holding that the causes of poverty lay in failures of individual character, COSs stood in unwavering opposition to public relief as condoning or even inducing pauperism (Ax-inn & Levin, 1997).

The first acknowledgment of government responsibility for family wel-fare appeared with the enactment of *mothers' pensions*, cash relief for wid-ows with children, beginning in 1911. Within 10 years, 40 states had developed such programs. At the federal level, the only relief programs were for federal employees and veterans and their families. Overall, pub-lic expenditures were meager: In 1913, the total amount of public relief at all levels was only 1% of total government expenditures (Axinn & Levin, 1997, p. 144). Local-level administrators, with offices characterized by "in-efficiency, political favoritism, and occasional fraud" (Steiner, 1966, p. 16) decided who would receive public assistance (Handler & Hasenfeld, 1991).

The Great Depression quickly overwhelmed both local coffers and vol-untary charity capacities, but the federal government was unwilling to re-spond readily despite clear signs of global distress. State disbursement of relief funds began in 1931, two years before the first federal relief effort, charged to the Federal Emergency Relief Administration (FERA). FERA channeled funds for cash and work relief through state and local welfare offices, requiring that the administration be by public, not private, agen-cies. Yet the intent was not to sustain a public relief program, but to sus-tain those who were unemployed until employment could be found. Harry Hopkins, FERA's director and advisor to the president, put it unequivo-cally: "Our job is to see that the unemployed get relief, not to develop a great social work organization throughout the United States" (cited in Ax-inn & Levin, 1997, p. 184). Two years after FERA's creation, direct federal relief tapered off, and the emphasis shifted to public works projects.

The federal relief effort, however brief, had a lasting effect in supplant-ing that of private charities, which in any event had historically opposed direct relief altogether. The private sector role increasingly became defined as providing services not linked to financial need. For the next quarter cen-tury, "money was public; counseling services were private" (Steiner, 1966, p. 17). At the same time, large numbers of social workers moved from the private to the public sector positions opened by relief. They and other so-cial welfare workers at state and federal levels formed constituencies fa-voring the expansion of public services, embodied first through the programs created in the Social Security Act of 1935.

The most important of these programs for the history of welfare case management is Aid to Dependent Children (ADC); this would evolve into Aid to Families with Dependent Children (AFDC), the type of income as-sistance most equated in the popular mind with *welfare*.[3] A state-adminis-tered grant-in-aid program, ADC was intended to promote the welfare of dependent children, providing stipends on a per-child basis. Like the mothers' pensions it supplanted, ADC supported primarily white widows, although no formal regulations restricted payments to children of color or those of unmarried mothers. Local boards and workers determined eligibility for the program, leading to great variability within and between states in policy and practice.

While the next three decades witnessed steady, or even apparently uncontrollable, growth in ADC rolls and expenditures,[4] the program itself changed only in incremental measure. Then, in 1962, the Public Welfare Amendments to the Social Security Act expanded on earlier changes to ADC, in the process opening the program to new recipients, services, and modes of service delivery. Renamed *Aid and Services to Needy Families with Children*, the program was henceforth referred to as *Aid to Families with Dependent Children* (AFDC). AFDC now included payments to unemployed parents and other "caretakers." It introduced and encouraged states to provide "preventive" and "rehabilitation" services aimed broadly at public welfare problems such as "dependency, juvenile delinquency, family breakdown, illegitimacy, ill health, and disability" (Axinn & Levin, 1997, pp. 238–241).[5] The introduction of these services initiated as well a new partnership between public welfare and nonprofit social welfare agencies, which could be contracted for social service delivery. The federal share of AFDC payments increased from 50 to 75% for states adopting the service approach fostered by these so-called Social Service Amendments, which also increased the federal share of payments to adult categories of recipients. Left untouched, however, was the overall philosophy and structure of state control over the administration of the program.

The social service approach would have a short life, culminating in the 1967 Amendments to the Social Security Act, referred to as Title IV-A. Born out of a mandated review of the 1962 provisions, Title IV-A embodied the recognition that the service approach had failed to prevent or reduce welfare dependency. Welfare rolls had continued to increase, with close to 1.5 times as many recipients in 1967 as in 1962, and federal costs were projected to increase by $26 billion over the next five years (Steiner, 1971). With program experts acknowledging that "You cannot casework poor people out of poverty" (quoted in Steiner, 1971, p. 25), Congress searched for other means to move people off the rolls and reduce expenditures, and found them in work incentives. The Work Incentive Program, "eventually known as WIN, after having initially and disastrously been referred to as WIP" (Axinn & Levin, 1997, p. 247), required employment or work training of adult AFDC recipients, offering incentives of day care funding and the "30/one-third" formula that let recipients keep the first thirty dollars and subsequent one-third of their wages before losing financial assistance. WIN was a harbinger of permanent change in welfare policy direction, promoting various combinations of work requirements and incentives in both state and federal programs.

Further indicating this shifting policy climate, the Department of Health, Education, and Welfare (HEW) restructured the administration of policy assistance, placing it within an agency headed by the former commissioner of the Vocational Rehabilitation Administration. While titling this the Social and Rehabilitation Service, HEW expected the new agency to de-emphasize social services in favor of rehabilitation services that were, in essence, work-oriented (Axinn & Levin, 1997). Administratively, services were "divorced" from assistance payments (Steiner, 1971, p. 25), announcing the intention that AFDC recipients would no longer automatically be required to receive social services. Favored by states for its potential cost savings and by social work professionals as enhancing both client rights and professional effectiveness, the administrative separation of financial assistance from social services became federal mandate by 1974.

While both Congress and HEW thus moved welfare away from the social service approach, they did not eliminate the provision of social services; in fact, it was acknowledged that such services were essential to making employment or work training viable. Title IV-A even broadened the language used to define services that could be given as well as who could receive them. The amendments also changed the way such services were to be provided, however, by authorizing the purchase of social services from private agencies through state contracts. This "purchase-of-service" mechanism had been foreseen in the original Social Security legislation (cf. Axinn & Levin, 1997), but had not been widely operational until this point. The new emphasis drew support from conservatives attempting to contain the rapidly expanding costs of public welfare, as well as from liberals using a politically feasible means to augment the reach and scope of public assistance.

Together, work incentive programs, separation of income maintenance, and purchase of service arrangements increased the administrative options open to state welfare programs, while transferring more service costs to the federal coffers. Predictably, federal social service expenditures mushroomed, showing a sixfold increase from 1967 to 1972 (Smith & Stone, 1988). Moves by Congress to cap expenditure levels met with strident opposition from coalitions of private and public social welfare providers. Regulatory compromises came in the form of Title XX of the Social Security Act, legislated in 1974. Title XX tightened the fiscal accountability required of states, but further expanded the definitions of service goals and potential recipients. It also increased the types and numbers of services delivered through contracts with both nonprofit and proprietary agencies.[6]

By the end of the 1970s, the division of social welfare was much as it was almost 50 years earlier: Money was public, services were private. Now the money was not only that provided to welfare recipients, but also that with which the government, still a reluctant provider, bought services from private sources. States had adopted an array of work incentive programs and ill-defined service commitments in the face of increasing economic stringency. Private and public agencies formed corporatist alliances shaping social policy and service delivery—and opposing reductions in funding. Social welfare had assumed a kaleidoscope image, its fragmented pieces reshaped to the politics and needs of each state and locale. Case management would be looked to as a way of reordering this picture and resolving the contradictions it contained.

WORK, WORTH, AND DESPAIR: SOCIETAL IMAGES OF THE WELFARE RECIPIENT

The evolution of welfare policy is, in large part, the process of creating and revising the moral classifications of the poor. (Handler & Hasenfeld, 1991, p. 37)

Public perceptions about what "the problem" is and moral constructions about how we should respond represent key dimensions of the social images attached to welfare and its recipients (Rochefort, 1986). Social images operate in several ways to affect welfare policy: They provide the basis for political rhetoric; they feed public sentiment and support; and they reinforce dominant social values such as those attached to work, the family, and social relations. These symbolic consequences can pertain regardless of the more objective outcomes of welfare policy. Public perceptions and moral constructions are thus not simply symbolic representations, but are also forces actively shaping the social reality of welfare practice (Handler & Hasenfeld, 1991).

One of the most potent of such forces in the history of social welfare in the United States has been the idea that not all poor people deserve state support. The point of moral categorization thus becomes separating the "deserving" from the "undeserving" poor (Handler & Hasenfeld, 1991). Dating back at least to the English Poor Law of 1601, the determination of deservingness centers on the question of individual responsibility: Is the person's character or behavior the source of the problem, or does it lie beyond the control of the individual (Rochefort, 1986)? Closely related are the principles of the Protestant work ethic with its emphasis on labor, discipline, and individual effort as yardsticks against which worthiness is measured (Handler & Hasenfeld, 1991; cf. Katz, 1986).

Starting in the 18th century, democratic politics and industrialization began to add a changed definition of *dependency* to concepts of worthiness and the work ethic as core principles of social welfare. Formerly, dependency connoted a subordinate position in a system of social relations and, as the normal and normative situation for most people, was morally neutral. As being *independent* came to imply a free citizen engaged in wage labor, dependency became a quality of the individual vested with pejorative moral and psychological meanings. Depending on charity relief instead of wage labor denoted one a pauper whose fate arose from immoral behavior or defects of character (Fraser & Gordon, 1994).

In the latter half of the 19th century, organized charities, and especially the Charity Organization Movement, elaborated concerns about pauperism within a framework of social Darwinism. In this view, the character defects of paupers were socially transmittable, if not biologically inherited. Public relief could thus promote degeneracy across generations unless it addressed the underlying basis of dependency in the indolent character. Tests of the ability to work and work requirements became the administrative routine and ideological core of both public and private relief.

Similar views of dependency emerged with justifications of colonial domination and slavery which linked subjugation to innate or characterological traits of the "natives" or slaves that made them dependent, "childlike," or "submissive" (Fraser & Gordon, 1994, p. 317). This racist discourse reinforced the image of dependency as a psychological property of a deviant group of individuals, rather than structural and political in origin. It also secured racialist thinking an essential place in reasoning about dependent populations.

Dependency had not yet assumed completely stigmatizing connotations, however. There remained a good form, that of wives and children dependent on a male wage earner. Based on labor's ideal of a wage adequate to support a family as well as the romanticization of homelife known as the *domestic code*, the model of household dependency held sway by the end of the 19th century. The dependency of housewives and children remained beyond the achievement of most families and more a cultural ideal than a generator of social policy until the Progressive era, when it became a cornerstone of the mothers' pension movement.

The grounding of mothers' pensions in principles of dependency and deservingness is clear in recommendations from the first White House Conference on Dependency in Children (which laid the principles for subsequent state action): "Children of reasonably efficient and deserving mothers who are without the support of the normal breadwinner should, as a rule be kept with their parents, such aid being given as may be necessary to maintain suitable homes for the rearing of children" (Bell, 1965, p. 4, quoted in Handler & Hasenfeld, 1991, p. 66). "Suitable homes" implied, in general, one with the mother at home caring for children full-time. Debates in advance of state pension legislation focused, however, on the moral perils of supporting deserted families or women with illegitimate children. Some in the organized charities felt, as well, that it would be better for mothers to work part-time since "life [at home] can be too dull sometimes" (Axinn & Levin, 1997, p. 142).

The way the pensions were enacted made the linkage of worth to work even more explicit. While the policy intent may have been to provide enough support that mothers need not work, the meager allocations made to the programs seldom left them any option. Moreover, while statutory coverage in many states extended to divorced, deserted, and unwed mothers, the actual recipients were overwhelmingly white widows; those whose male breadwinner was absent involuntarily (Handler & Hasenfeld, 1991).

Despite their greater reach, New Deal relief programs continued to reflect traditional views of work, worth, and dependency. No less a player than President Roosevelt himself voiced apprehensions that "continued dependence on relief induces a spiritual and moral disintegration fundamentally destructive to the national fibre" (Katz, 1986, p. 226). Reinforced by concern in the business community about labor discipline, this stance ensured that the New Deal's programs for the unemployed offered primarily menial jobs with low wages, available only to those who passed means tests.[7]

The Social Security Act of 1935 created a two-track welfare system that concretized the principles and inequalities of its predecessors. First-track programs such as unemployment and old age insurance operated as specially funded entitlements aimed at replacement of the family wage. For at least their first three decades, their primary recipients were white male laborers, and the assumptions built into their structure continue to work against those whose labor patterns differ from that group, including most women and minorities (Gordon, 1994; Rodeheaver, 1987). Aid to Dependent Children (ADC) became the most visible of the second-track programs, which ran on general revenues distributed to recipients through means-testing. While its statutory coverage was less restrictive than the older state mothers' aid programs, the administration of ADC continued to rely on "morals-testing" (Fraser & Gordon, 1994, p. 322) to sort out the deserving. Policies requiring recipients to demonstrate their "fitness" to raise children in "suitable" homes translated in practice to the virtual exclusion from benefits of unwed mothers and women of color (Axinn & Levin, 1997, pp. 191–192). Rules against having an unrelated "man in the house" built on the same moral criteria, elaborating as well the ideology excluding potential male labor from relief rolls (Piven & Cloward, 1993). Caseworkers conducted intensive surveillance of recipients' home lives, using findings of "unsuitability" or the presence at midnight of an unrelated man to close cases. While court and executive rulings eventually end-

ed such exclusions, their importance lay as well in the changes they sig-
naled in social perceptions of welfare recipients. The overall cast of ADC
stigmatized even the "worthy" recipients, who suffered from demeaning
administrative measures and the assumption that they were getting a free
ride at the public's expense.

At the same time, and at least in theory, several provisions of the Social
Security Act removed welfare forever from the traditional relief programs
epitomized in the almshouse and moved toward the idea of a "right to assistance" (Axinn & Levin, 1997, p. 190). These provisions included the definition of assistance as cash grants, the requirement that recipients live in
their own homes, and mandates for a fair hearing for individuals denied a
claim. In the decades following World War II, welfare rights activists would
convert the idea of a right to aid into a substantial liberalization of ADC.

From the mid-1950s through the end of the 1960s, demographic, economic, political, and intellectual trends converged to reinforce negative
images of public assistance and its recipients. Exponential increases in welfare rolls at a time of general prosperity implied to many that the social de-
viance of recipients accounted for their separation from the job market. In
1961, the Secretary of Health, Education, and Welfare (HEW) expressed
concern about the "second and third generation of people on relief"; later
in the decade, Daniel Patrick Moynihan would point to "the development
of a permanently dependent class" as the source of the welfare "crisis"
(Rochefort, 1986, p. 103). Culture of poverty theories arose to account for
this entrenched dependency. At the core of models looking at poverty as
the result of pathology were psychological and behavioral traits thought
distinctive of poor people: Even when these theories acknowledged social
problems such as segregation and discrimination as root causes, they never moved far from a view of poverty as individual pathology (Rochefort,
1986; Handler & Hasenfeld, 1991).

By the early 1970s, negative views of welfare dependency deepened as
women began entering the labor force in greater numbers. In addition,
white women were increasingly covered under social insurance programs—unemployment, survivors insurance—which did not have the
same stigma as welfare, which in turn became associated increasingly with
racial minorities. Public opinion began to reveal a backlash against welfare
clients, who were seen as deceptive manipulators of the system who had
children to get benefits (Rochefort, 1986). Reflecting the increased call to
sort out the worthy, the 1967 amendments cut payments for cases of de-
sertion and illegitimacy and initiated work requirements.

Deservingness, the work ethic, and dependency have been a symbolic
triad, constantly threading through welfare policy. Reinforced by views of
women, people of color, family roles, and class relations, these images have
been ways of identifying worth, linking it to work, and reinforcing the

"right" dependency, namely, on work or on men. As the welfare rolls exploded from the late 1960s on, these images increasingly moved the system away from a view of welfare rights and toward a model expecting much of welfare recipients, while still stigmatizing them.

THE "ALBATROSS OF RELIEF" AND THE
PROFESSION OF SOCIAL WORK

As a profession, social work considers social welfare its domain, and indeed its early development as a profession is inseparable from the welfare movements of the Progressive era. Seen historically, however, the relationship of the profession to public welfare is also one of conflict. Opposed to public relief, its member association attempts to make social casework the cornerstone of welfare services, all the while excluding from its ranks the majority of public welfare workers. Attempts by leaders of the profession to increase the standards for welfare casework backfire in the lowering of requirements for a public social worker position. Public assistance casework embodies contradictory principles of social reform and social control, centered on sorting the worthy from unworthy recipients and monitoring their continued worthiness. These dynamics would lead social work to promote the introduction of case management in the welfare domain, while making relations between case managers and clients inherently ambivalent.

Professional social work evolved from the efforts of 19th century reformers leading the settlement house and Charity Organization movements. Charity Organization Societies (COSs), which would come to dominate social welfare past the turn of the century, operated under the philosophy that relief should be limited, provided only after careful investigation, and linked to work. Their "friendly visitors," chiefly well-to-do women, set out to help the poor "find social and economic salvation through work" and to "help the individual, through example and precept, through the sympathy and encouragement of personal relations, to rise above the need for relief" (Axinn & Levin, 1997, pp. 96–97). Though volunteers, these workers played essentially a casework role, winnowing out the undeserving and counseling recipients on how to lift themselves from poverty. By the 1920s, private relief agencies had replaced COSs, and paid workers replaced volunteers, but using largely the same techniques of social control and social reform. Mary Richmond, a leader in the COS movement, codified these precepts into treatises on social casework published in 1917 and 1922, initiating "a therapeutic model of professional service" (Axinn & Levin, 1997, p. 149) that was shortly embedded in the first social work training programs.

The Great Depression was a watershed for the role and orientation of the profession. Social work professionals were key to the development of the public welfare sphere as the private sector found itself unable to respond to the extent of relief required. Many social workers were active in social reform and community organizing, and private agencies lent staff to public service, provided aid in supervision and consultation, and roused public support for relief. When federal regulations required that relief funds be administered by public agencies, the private agency workers became public officials, bringing with them a "professional casework service orientation toward relief giving" (Axinn & Levin, 1997, p. 186). Caseworkers had enormous discretion in determining eligibility, the level and form of support, and which aspects of recipients' lives were pertinent to their cases.

By the 1950s, social workers were at the center of public welfare, holding administrative positions at all levels. The frontline assistance workers tended to be individuals with baccalaureate or less training, however. In the midst of efforts to control the licensing and certification of workers, social work leadership founded the National Association of Social Workers (NASW) in 1955.[8] NASW saw public assistance as a stumbling block on its path to increased professional status, and both the association and public assistance administrators pushed to increase the number of trained social work graduates in public service.

In 1961, the Secretary of HEW appointed an almost all social work ad hoc committee that would be the architect of the Public Welfare Amendments of 1962, the social service amendments that would mark the waxing of social work's professional influence within public assistance. The committee held objectives that were hallmarks of a social casework approach: that one-third of all public welfare social workers would be at MSW level, that caseloads would not exceed 60 recipients per worker, that there would be a 1:5 supervisory ratio, and that workers would engage in frequent home visiting. The social services themselves consisted mainly of casework (and later, case management) practice, including assessment, individualized service plans, information-giving, advice, and referral to other community agencies, with 75% of costs reimbursed to states by the federal government (Steiner, 1966; Marmor & Rein, 1973).

Supporters of the social service approach held forth expectations that as recipients achieved independence, there would be benefits for both family well-being and the public coffers. As these results did not appear, even in carefully designed projects comparing routine casework with intensive services by professional workers (Steiner, 1971), social work's professional influence began to wane. Other disciplines, such as political science and economics, began asserting their expertise on issues of poverty and welfare, critiquing the social casework approach as "patronizing and intrusive" (Rochefort, 1986, p. 111). The criticism had certainly been warranted by casework practices translating "suitable home" and "man in the house" rulings into punitive and exclusionary actions. While executive and court rulings abolished the worst of these measures, groups claiming to represent welfare recipients, such as the National Welfare Rights Organization, joined the criticism of social work's control over welfare administration. In shifting from a social service to a work program emphasis, the 1967 Social Security Amendments opened the door for further diminishment of the profession's role.

In the view of the profession, part of the blame for the failure of a social service approach lay in the fact that caseworkers still were not, by and large, trained social workers. Far from the ratio of one MSW to 60 cases envisioned in 1962, by one estimate roughly 4% of public assistance workers had such training (Steiner, 1971). Professional workers were instead being drawn to private agencies, and the production of new MSWs by schools of social work lagged far behind the need for staff occasioned by the ever-expanding rolls. The professional leadership saw removing income maintenance from casework as essential to drawing more trained workers to public employment, as well as making the service approach viable. In an editorial in the field's premiere journal, NASW leader Gordon Hamilton decried, "Social work to date has never been allowed the tools, even on a minimum level, to make public assistance a helping function. . . . Why not place the basic maintenance grant in a separate unit . . . and staff this unit with well trained civil servants? . . . Why not take the albatross of 'relief' . . . from the neck of social service?" (cited in Steiner, 1966, p. 185). The national association also favored separation on the grounds that it would reinforce a concept of assistance as a right rather than conditional on service participation, would promote clients' "self-determination in seeking and accepting service" (Axinn & Levin, 1997, p. 248), and would permit better targeting of services to those needing them—all goals consistent with professional objectives.

Separation would not, however, lead to the advancement of professional social work within the public sector. By the late 1970s, surveys on the qualifications of public welfare personnel found the majority of states reporting that they made no distinction between workers trained in social work (at BSW or MSW levels) and others in hiring direct service workers, or in promoting them as supervisors (Wyers, 1980; Pecora & Austin, 1983).

Separation also did not appear to achieve the other goals held by the profession. State offices increased caseloads for financial assistance workers (in places, more than doubling them), while neither workers nor clients were certain how the labor was being divided. Research findings showed recipients requesting services less and seeing case workers as less helpful under the new arrangement than the old one, rating them on average only slightly above the midpoint on a scale from "not at all" to "very helpful" (Piliavin & Gross, 1977). One financial worker described the strain on his end:

> We were now forced by our higher caseloads to refer most service needs to the service units. Even so, many of our referrals were held up because of a lack of direction or policy in the Social Service units, the system being so new. The clients still called us for help with their family problems . . . workers began to quit the Department and absenteeism increased greatly. Also, workers began to "go into the field" in the afternoon to escape, rather than to work. They slammed down phones quite frequently and "blew up" in the office. The phones were constantly ringing, grating upon everyone's nerves. Workers began to take tranquilizers frequently. Five milligrams of Valium was the dosage commonly used. Some workers withdrew to the roof and smoked marijuana, but returned to discover themselves even more jittery. (Greenblatt & Richmond, 1979, pp. 10–11)

During the latter half of the 1970s, civil service reforms and antidiscrimination rulings combined with paraprofessional staff development programs in a development further threatening the status of professional social work within social welfare. Termed *reclassification* by proponents and *declassification* by its foes, this trend involved efforts by state civil service commissions to ease educational job restrictions by reducing educational requirements for entry-level positions, equating experience with education for advancement, and considering equivalent all baccalaureate-level training, regardless of field. In addition, the identity of the public sector social worker was being further eroded as states formed large umbrella human service bureaucracies, generally managed by non-social work administrators who failed to see a need for specialized training for social service delivery (Pecora & Austin, 1983).

These trends involved big stakes numerically, since by some estimates half of over 800,000 human service workers in the country had positions titled "social workers"; and over 80% of the social work labor force was employed in public agencies. In fighting reclassification, NASW found itself at odds with the American Federation of State, County, and Municipal Employees (AFSCME), the union representing the majority of the 15 to 20% of human service social workers who were unionized (Karger, 1983). The stakes here were clearly more than numeric, since the standards and role of the profession itself were in question. NASW continued to hold that "upper-level and key line personnel must have social work degrees; . . . social workers should direct and control public social services; . . . [and] there is no equivalent to a professional social work education" (Karger, 1983, p. 429).

Never completely comfortable with public relief, social work now faced profound threats to its influence and professional agenda in social welfare. NASW's strategic responses included public relations and educational campaigns on the value of social work, as well as technical assistance to chapters in states undergoing reclassification (Karger, 1983). Given the broader antiwelfare sentiment of the time, and the pressures on states accruing from new federalism, these responses hardly seemed adequate. A new vehicle was essential for the casework approach to remain part of public welfare.

WELFARE, WORK, AND CASE MANAGEMENT

We have seen how the pluralistic organization of social welfare, social images of deservingness and dependency, and professional dynamics acted as intertwined threads giving shape to welfare policy as it evolved in the 20th century. The ties among those threads would tighten as AFDC became increasingly focused on welfare-to-work programs in the 1970s and 1980s. Bearing increased fiscal loads of multifaceted programs, government authorities looked for administrative mechanisms that could coordinate services and save costs. Changes in social images created the perception of welfare recipients as multiproblem individuals in need of multiple service solutions; these changes also multiplied the voices claiming the welfare experience as their domain and extended the distance between recipients and providers. Social workers and related social welfare groups tried to counteract the deprofessionalization of welfare workers and maintain professional influence over the definition of welfare services. Case management became part of welfare-to-work programs toward the end of the 1970s in response to the challenges and opportunities the linkages among these trends created.

In the broader domain of social welfare and antipoverty programs, case management had already become well established as part of the technology of service coordination efforts (Kagan & Neville, 1993; National Conference on Social Welfare, 1977). The cornerstone of President Johnson's War on Poverty, Community Action Agencies (CAAs) used case management as one among many planning and linking mechanisms to coordinate local-level projects. Services Integration Targets of Opportunity (SITO) projects succeeded CAAs in the early 1970s as a method of consolidating and coordinating human services. Designed as research and demonstration programs to provide data about the process and outcomes of service integration, SITO projects included case managers among other systems integration devices such as client pathways, service taxonomies, and internal performance measures. Case management next found its place among 10 management elements as part of research and demonstration programs in the Comprehensive Human Services Planning and Delivery System (CHSPDS) projects, beginning in 1975. Succeeding CHSPDS in a final general focus on service coordination, the Service Integration Pilot Projects (SIPPs), starting in 1984, focused on needs-based services and goals of promoting self-sufficiency, which included lowering the number of welfare recipients. Again, a case management approach was central to these efforts.

Service integration efforts were closely tied to another trend that would more directly bring case management into welfare programs. From the latter half of the 1960s on, states assumed central control of welfare administration, in part to standardize payments and services, and in part to relieve the administrative burdens of smaller local districts (Greenblatt & Richmond, 1979). Although states and local programs no longer controlled categorical eligibility, they still set standards for financial eligibility and benefit levels. This enabled them to clamp down on expenditures even as AFDC rolls skyrocketed.[9] The Work Incentive programs (now termed *WIN*) remained relatively uniform across states with AFDC requirements that recipients register and participate or face termination or reductions of grants.

President Reagan's administration inaugurated a further shift of welfare responsibility to the states with the Omnibus Budget Reconciliation Act (OBRA) of 1981. OBRA permitted the states several options for programs with work requirements that, although providing more AFDC administrative monies, required greater commitment of state matching funds. On net, due to program shifts and budgetary cuts in funding of WIN, OBRA resulted in state welfare programs scrambling to organize new programs. Their attempts were further complicated by the continued national economic malaise as well as the reductions in federal funding that came with Social Service Block Grants (Handler & Hasenfeld, 1991; Stone & Smith, 1988). Ironically, the number and diversity of programs involved with welfare offices continued to multiply as contracting with private agencies, not only for direct services but in some cases for administrative functions, became a key survival strategy in this context (Smith & Stone, 1988; Smith & Lipsky, 1993).

Social images of the welfare population continued to build on the negative perceptions of earlier decades, elaborating now an ideology that welfare should be provided only for the "truly needy" while those who could work, should do so (Handler & Hasenfeld, 1991, 170). At the same time, perceptions of other problems and populations became increasingly liberal during this period. Lay and professional interests prompted the "discovery" and treatment as social problems of a variety of formerly individual troubles, including domestic violence, learning disabilities, and alcohol and substance abuse. *Dependency* and *codependency* became pathological categories scrutinized in academic research as well as popular media (Fraser & Gordon, 1994). Groups already categorically recognized as dependent in medical and legal parlance began to contest the form of their recognition and treatment; key here are consumer movements among those with physical disability and mental illness.

These events reverberated in public welfare in two ways. First, they provided a new discourse for characterizing the welfare population; as concerns about welfare dependency mounted, the reasons for that dependency could now be sought in an increasing array of individual and family pathologies.[10] Developments parallel to consumer movements provided, as well, a discourse of resistance, as groups of welfare recipients sought more client-centered programs. Second, accompanying the elaboration of social problems was an ever-expanding roster of programs providing diagnosis and treatment of individual cases. These would, at least hypothetically, be among the noneconomic services needed to help welfare recipients achieve personal and economic independence, or at least employment—increasingly the primary goals of welfare policy.

Adopting those goals also involved administrative changes that further complicated the welfare system and challenged the professionalism of its workers. Separate state agencies became linked to WIN programs and subsequent demonstrations, as AFDC recipients received vocational rehabilitation, child care, food stamps, and a variety of social services (including those of child welfare offices). AFDC frontline staff became "integrated generalists" dealing with very mixed caseloads and doing all casework functions (Greenblatt & Richmond, 1979). Requirements that caseworkers document all changes in recipients' income, expenses, family composition, and other circumstances intensified under OBRA's provisions. There had already been growing attention to the use of management information systems and other forms of "management technology" within public social service programs, including the use of automated systems within case management for service planning and monitoring (National Conference on Social Welfare, 1976). By the early 1980s, state offices were applying automation to many aspects of AFDC work, and there was increased administrative focus on error control, with severe federal penalties placed on states whose error rates exceeded a certain level (Brodkin & Lipsky, 1983; Handler & Hasenfeld, 1991). At the worker level, these moves translated into increased paperwork and decreased discretion. An account by an assistance worker illustrates how computerization added to the workload while creating a new form of "bureaucratic disentitlement" (Lipsky, 1984; cf. Handler & Hasenfeld, 1991):

> A special person in the office worked on a computer print-out, seeking to find our clients among those on a list of clients receiving unemployment compensation. He gave us the names of the people who were collecting, and we had to call them in to close out or reduce their assistance. One print-out con-

tained the names of people to whom the Department had sent letters but whose letters had been returned to us; we were ordered to close the cases. When we sent out routine letters and they were returned, addressee unknown, we were ordered to close these cases also. Many times, mail was returned in error, clients came in angry, and we had to re-open the case, a process requiring a ten-page re-application form. (Greenblatt & Richmond, 1979, p. 15)

These developments were of concern to organizations claiming to represent the interests of welfare workers, but it was unclear what an appropriate response would be. Case management had already come to the attention of the social welfare field, and it was becoming evident that case management would have a place in future welfare reform. By the late 1970s, case management had become a regular feature in various areas of social welfare, including child welfare and programs for the developmentally disabled (National Conference on Social Welfare, 1981; Zlotnik, 1996; Hegar, 1992). In a 1980 National Case Management Conference on developmental disabilities sponsored by the National Conference on Social Welfare (an interorganizational association that held an influential annual forum on social welfare issues), the question of staff professionalism found heated expression:

> The question of whether case managers should be professionals or para-professionals met with considerable controversy; in fact, opinions were about evenly divided. Many felt that a professional background was invaluable in providing the case manager with the authority and clout necessary to perform the job effectively. . . . While it was agreed that competent case managers could be drawn from any number of disciplines, social workers emerged as the most natural choice. Meanwhile, concern about overprofessionalizing the case management field was significant; many feared the development of a job description so rigorous and specialized that few could meet its requirements. The use of para-professionals was a popular alternative. (National Conference on Social Welfare, 1981, p. 6)

As welfare-to-work programs began to adopt case management, the extent of professionalism required for and of their staff would continue to be a contested issue.

MOVING TO JOBS: CASE MANAGEMENT
ENTERS PUBLIC WELFARE

By the mid-1980s, almost all states had started new programs centered on moving recipients off the rolls and into jobs. Program requirements ranged from subsidized on-the-job training to mandatory job search activities, to requiring participation in an unpaid job while on the rolls. These programs expanded in the late 1980s to include an even greater range of designs, types of coverage, and costs (Gueron, Pauly, & Lougy, 1991; Nightingale, Wissoker, Burbridge, Bawden, & Jeffries, 1991; Riccio, Goldman, Hamilton, Martinson, & Orenstein, 1989; Handler & Hasenfeld, 1991). In some, such as Massachusett's Employment and Training (ET), participation was essentially voluntary, and recipients had a choice of services. California's Greater Avenues for Independence (GAIN) and New Jersey's Realizing Economic Achievement (REACH) required participation in educational, training, and work programs as determined through a complex client assessment system.

In some programs, the welfare agency and the client signed a formal agreement outlining each party's responsibilities, seen in places as enforceable under state contract law. More generally, the new programs embodied a consensus that the role of government support was to provide incentives and services to help recipients obtain employment, while recipients assumed the responsibility of participating in employment services and taking jobs. In practice, this translated into increased emphasis on obtaining child support from noncustodial parents and on providing child care, education and training opportunities, and employment services such as job searches (Gueron et al., 1991). Some programs targeted particular groups of long-term welfare recipients, providing them with subsidized employment or with intensive, supervised work experience and on-the-job training (Ibid.; cf. Maynard, 1993; Hamilton, Burstein, Hargreaves, Moss, & Walker, 1993; Perlmutter, 1997). The increased diversity of service options and the targeting procedures needed to sort clients into appropriate pathways made these programs more complex administratively than previous welfare-to-work attempts.[11]

As this suggests, these new programs centered on case management, but they organized case management in different ways. While some relied on generalist case managers to handle everything for particular clients, others divided the tasks of assessment, monitoring, or brokering services between case managers and other staff, or even among different provider agencies. Case managers' job descriptions and caseload sizes varied accordingly (Gueron et al., 1991; Doolittle & Riccio, 1992).[12]

Evidence quickly mounted in support of the new programs' effectiveness, although outcomes appeared to hinge greatly on local economic and political conditions (Handler & Hasenfeld, 1991; O'Neill, 1990). Moreover, each design choice carried compromises in the objectives that could be achieved. One synthesis of research findings notes that low-cost, broad-coverage programs (requiring mainly job search activities) achieved "consistent and sustained increases in employment and earnings" and "relatively large welfare savings per dollar spent," but the gains came from increasing the number of people working, not improving job quality, so that many recipients remained in poverty (Gueron et al., 1991, p. 36). In contrast, targeted programs providing subsidized employment, more costly to begin with, yielded "consistent and sustained increases in employment and earnings" but "relatively small welfare savings per dollar spent" (Ibid.). Analyses of work-for-relief programs showed an even harsher concession: "Work programs . . . demonstrate that with strict enforcement and use of sanctions, adequate fiscal investment, and a requirement that the poor work for their welfare benefits if they cannot find jobs, it is possible to substitute work for welfare, especially if the concern to improve the economic well-being of the poor is abandoned" (Handler & Hasenfeld, 1991, pp. 185–186). Regardless of program design, costs and benefits for recipients inevitably faced a trade-off with those for taxpayers, limiting the extent to which programs achieving greatest results for recipients could also achieve long-term political support (Handler & Hasenfeld, 1991).

Notwithstanding these equivocal results, welfare reform came back to the national agenda in the second half of the 1980s with both conservatives and liberals supporting the welfare-to-work approach. Conservatives viewed the outcomes of state programs as proving that the poor could be moved into work, saving public money. Following the administration's lead, they favored measures increasingly shifting responsibility for the design and implementation of welfare-to-work programs to the states (Handler & Hasenfeld, 1991). Liberals, faced with the impossibility of increasing spending on social issues given the escalating national deficit, pushed to augment efforts preparing recipients for employment, such as literacy, remedial education, general equivalency diploma (GED), job readiness, and training programs (Noble, 1997).

The Family Support Act (FSA) of 1988 incorporated both conservative and liberal agendas, replacing WIN and other work programs with the Job Opportunities and Basic Skills (JOBS) program. JOBS placed responsibility on recipients to participate in employment services and to take jobs, and on the government to provide incentives and supports for this effort. While leaving the basic entitlement nature of AFDC intact, it made clear that welfare receipt was intended to be a "temporary support" rather than "permanent income maintenance" (Gueron et al., 1991, p. 1). FSA set mandates and incentives (in the form of new matching funds) for state action in welfare-to-work programs and, modeling JOBS broadly on the GAINS program, required that programs conduct assessments, develop "employability plans," and provide certain educational and job skills, readiness, development, and placement services as well as child care. JOBS targeted potentially long-term recipients and extended participation in work programs to all mothers whose youngest child was three or older; states could elect to include part-time work requirements for those with a youngest child older than one year. States had great latitude regarding exemptions, however, and participation was expected to increase incrementally, with the mandate that 20% of nonexempt eligible recipients be enrolled by 1995. The legislation and subsequent regulations also provided only a broad framework for JOBS program design, leaving most operational decisions up to the states (Handler & Hasenfeld, 1991; Noble, 1997).

FSA designated case management an optional feature of a state's JOBS program. The Final Regulations implementing the law spelled out very little about the nature or requirements of this feature; in their entirety, they stipulate: "(a) the State IV-A agency may assign a case manager to a participant and the participant's family. The decision to assign a case manager may be made on a case-by-case basis. (b) The case manager must be responsible for assisting the family to obtain any services that may be needed to assure effective participation in the program" (Federal Register, 1989, section 250.43, p. 42179).

PROFESSIONAL HOPES AND CASE MANAGEMENT REALITIES

The JOBS mandate for case management was clearly less than had been hoped for by some parties representing social welfare workers. The American Public Welfare Association (APWA), the national organization of state and local public welfare departments, had issued a report on childhood poverty two years earlier calling for a "case management system in all human service agencies to help families assess their needs and resources and to implement and monitor the agency-client contract" (cited in APWA, 1993, p. 4). In 1987, APWA proposed a welfare reform plan with case management as a "key component" (cited in Doolittle & Riccio, 1992, p. 310). Reflecting the interests of its membership, which included semiprofessional welfare workers in addition to administrators, APWA recommended that states require at least an associate degree, and eventually a bachelor's degree, for case managers. In a statement presented at the hearings of a subcommittee of the Senate Finance Committee on the bill that would become FSA, APWA officials again pressed for case management in "all public human service agencies" to "brok[er] and coordinat[e] the social, health, education, and employment services necessary to promote self-sufficiency and strengthen families" (Testimony of Stephen B. Heintz . . . , 1987, p. 8). One of seven key elements of APWA's proposal for a Family Investment Program, the envisioned case management approach was both broad and intensive, encompassing "all of the 'needs' that relate to both self-sufficiency options and the strength and stability of the family unit . . ." (Ibid., p. 12).

NASW also continued to press its casework agenda. At the same hearings, the association's president asserted the need for "outreach, counseling, case management, and other services which equip people socially, psychologically, and emotionally to succeed in work and training programs" as essential elements for "any effort at meaningful welfare reform . . ." (U.S. Senate Committee on Finance, S. Hrg 100–335, 1987, p. 351). Other sources make it clear that the association still intended this case management to be delivered by personnel with higher professional qualifications. Surveying the deprofessionalization of case management throughout the social services over the past decade, the NASW Delegate Assembly of 1987 approved a policy statement attesting: "It is our obligation to our clients to arrest a movement that deprives clients of professional psychosocial assessment, skilled counseling, mediating interventions with service providers at each stage of the process, and advocacy efforts that will increase clients' options. . . . NASW strongly urges the use of professional social workers in all aspects of the delivery of case management services" (NASW, 1997, pp. 42–43).

Though APWA and NASW were both promoting case management, the tenor of their support reflected different underlying philosophies about how case management would serve family support objectives. For APWA, the emphasis was on service contracts and the assumption of individual responsibility. NASW's approach, to use its own terminology, was "softer," involving holistic support for families in line with a casework modality. These reflected, respectively, norms of social control and of social reform that had always been uncomfortably conjoined in public welfare and that would continue to be reflected in case management practice.

Responding to pressures to make case management mandatory and/or specify the types and levels of training in the description of case management programs, the Family Support Administration rules made clear the ideological underpinnings of the FSA approach: "We . . . realize that there are reasons that a State may not use case management or use it only in certain instances. Cost may be one such reason. We believe that each State can best decide the proper utilization of case management for the needs of that state. . . . [W]e decline to mandate that specific features of case management be adopted or that case managers be required to receive specified training. We leave these matters to the discretion of the States" (Federal Register, 1989, section 250.43, p. 42180). Notwithstanding APWA's and NASW's desire for a more expansive system, it would have to suffice that JOBS shifted public welfare from a system "that emphasizes income support and fiscal accuracy to one that emphasizes the delivery of services" (Hagen, 1994, p. 197), as noted by an evaluator of JOBS program implementation in NASW's leading journal. She and other observers felt the emphasis on services and case management was a good indication that "states are struggling to get welfare officials to act more like social workers and less like accountants" (Kosterlitz, 1989, quoted in Hagen op cit.).

It was not easy to see that struggle in the structure of early JOBS case management efforts, however. Case managers were predominantly staff already present in welfare offices, and the vast majority had baccalaureate- or lower-level education (Hagen & Lurie, 1994a, b; APWA, 1992). Only Mississippi required that case managers be licensed social workers.[13] The role of JOBS case managers was predominantly that of a service broker, since most of the educational and employment services from other providers were not reimbursed under JOBS. Neither were supportive services such as counseling, family planning, or substance abuse treatment made features of the assessment process or service referrals in JOBS in most states (Hagen & Lurie, 1994a). Case managers thus depended on the availability of community services and the cooperation of other agencies to meet client needs. In early surveys most case managers reported being hampered in their broker efforts by inadequate funding of education, employment and training services, as well as insufficient employment opportunities (Hagen & Lurie, 1994a, b; APWA, 1993).

Internal resources were also problematic: Initially, states were not spending enough of their funds to get all their federal entitlement of JOBS funds, and some experienced chronic underfunding (Hagen & Lurie, 1994a). Some states responded by cuts in staff; Massachusetts, for example, cut the number of case managers in MassJOBS to less than half of what it had been in ET (SEIU Local 509, n.d.). Ironically, in an effort to achieve better internal coordination, some states reunited income assistance with social service functions under case managers (Hagen & Lurie, 1994a).

Another issue restricting case managers was the size of their caseloads. Few states restricted them; surveys found they averaged above 100, with case managers in some states reporting over 250 or even 500 cases (APWA, 1993; Hagen & Lurie, 1994a). Bottlenecks in registering clients in JOBS developed as the overall caseloads in AFDC kept rising. Caseloads this size limited case managers' ability to work individually with clients, and one survey found one-third of their work time taken by required data entry and paperwork (Hagen & Lurie, 1994a.). Together with the emphasis on tracking and monitoring clients' participation in service programs (mandated federally on the grounds that it would reduce "no-shows" and program dropouts), the clerical nature of case managers' work reportedly made them feel like "simply caseworkers" (Hagen & Lurie, op. cit., p. 12). Monitoring activities also complicated relationships with clients, since persistent noncompliance with the program plan could lead to the financial sanction of a grant reduction.

Given that the case manager role in JOBS was "primarily that of a broker of services, at best, and . . . a monitor of client participation" (Hagen &

Lurie, op. cit., p. xi), some analysts felt "it may be more accurate to call these types of positions case maintenance or case monitoring rather than case management" (Ibid.). Certainly case managers had far less than the education, training, supervisory support, and program control the APWA and NASW had envisioned as key to their performance.

JOBS: CASE MANAGEMENT IN PRACTICE

On paper, case management in the JOBS program looks much like its counterparts in other sectors. Its basic functions include assessment, service planning, service implementation, and monitoring; secondary functions sometimes include advocacy, counseling, and follow-up after a case is closed. In dealing with clients, many of whom have physical, emotional, behavioral, and family problems complicating their situations, case managers attempt to work from a holistic perspective on both needs and strengths of clients and their families. And the models of case management services include generalist, specialist, and team approaches, as described subsequently (APWA, 1993, 1994).

As was the case for mental health, JOBS case management came out of a national policy initiative implemented under the control of state- and local-level agencies. The structure and operations of case management programs thus show incredible variability. Among the few constants across sites are chronic resource shortages, increasing caseloads, and the reliance on services acquired by referral rather than purchase (Hagen & Lurie, 1994a, b).

There are, however, important differences between JOBS case management and that in other sectors. First is that the paramount goal of the program is to move clients out of the system; that is, get them off of welfare and into employment. Case management here is therefore somewhat like hospital discharge planning, formulating a plan and timetable for closing the case from its beginning at intake (APWA, 1993). The plan, moreover, is based on a contractual agreement with the client, and case managers have at their disposal sanctions for enforcing the contract. The use of contracts and sanctions complicates the role of case manager here above and beyond its usual complexities (Hasenfeld & Weaver, 1996.). In addition, JOBS case managers are less likely to have professional degrees than those in other fields; they are also more likely to work within a highly bureaucratized agency.

In all, JOBS case management programs operate in the midst of contradictions. They have the impetus of policy objectives with broad national support, but what they actually do varies from one town to the next. They attempt to decrease welfare dependency, but their efforts are hindered by social images stereotyping such dependency as well as recipients. They

model themselves as a professional service based on frontline worker discretion, but must perform in a bureaucratic context where formal regulations prevail.

The following sections show how these contradictions are apparent in
the contexts in which case managers work and in their relations with welfare recipients. While there has been less examination of case management
practice than its outcomes, several studies have provided systematic
analyses of how JOBS case management works, differences among programs, and participant reactions (Hagen & Lurie, 1994a, b; APWA, 1992,
1993; Hasenfeld & Weaver, 1996). Supplementing those findings are case
materials that emerged in my research on case management in the JOBS
program in Massachusetts (MassJOBS), which was conducted in collaboration with David Rochefort of Northeastern University.[14]

Local-Level Variation, or When to Call
the Ukrainian Restaurant

Given the history of public welfare, it is not surprising to find differences
among JOBS programs in the structure and activities of case management.
Surveys across the states have identified three basic case management
models: the generalist model in which clients are assigned to one particular case manager who is responsible for all phases of their participation in
the program; the specialist approach, which assigns particular phases
(such as initial appraisal), activities (such as career counseling), or service
connections (such as job development) to workers with specialist training;
and a team model combining specialists from different program components or service providers (APWA, 1993;cf. Hargreaves, 1993). One study
covering all the states, the District of Columbia, and two territories found
generalist models were most common (found in 70% of sites); the specialist approach and team case management were also highly developed
(found in 5 and 7 states, respectively; APWA, 1992). State and local programs also show high variability in the caseload assigned to case managers. The majority (64%) in the APWA survey were found to have set
maximum caseload standards, but of those which had, standards ranged
from 35 to 325 (with an average of 98), while actual caseloads ranged from
10 to 500 with an average of 118. The organizational location for JOBS case
management has most commonly been a public welfare department, but
has also included other governmental offices as well as private agencies
working on contract. Supervisory structures and ratios have also varied,
as do the background required for case managers; while most programs
have required at least an associate or bachelor's degree, slightly more than
one-third have had no educational requirement beyond high school, and
only 60% mandated some professional experience (APWA, 1994).

In addition to these differences in formal structure, JOBS programs have varied in their operating philosophies, goals, and service technologies (Hasenfeld & Weaver, 1996; Handler & Hasenfeld, 1991). Differences in philosophy include the perspective used to understand why recipients are on welfare; for example, whether they are seen as deficient in their work ethic *versus* lacking education, training, or opportunity. Program goals vary from that of immediate job placement to an emphasis on long-term human capital investments. Service technologies vary in the extent to which bureaucratic rules, professional judgment, or moral evaluation provides the basis for decision making. The choice of philosophy, goals, and technology represents a program's strategic adaptation to its local political economy and service community, and these elements in turn shape relationships with clients and the means used to deal with noncompliance (Hasenfeld & Weaver, 1996).

What difference do these formal and informal program differences make? Evaluations of JOBS programs and their predecessor welfare-to-work demonstrations have failed to find systematic disparities on performance or outcome measures among programs differing by type or structure. Thus, there appears to be no one best model of case management, set of staff qualifications or training, supervisory approach, job performance assessment criteria, or caseload size.[15] Caseload size, or case management "intensity," has been a variable particularly of concern for the JOBS program given suggestions in the literature that more "intense" relations between case managers and participants could promote better outcomes. A demonstration in Riverside, California, attempted to evaluate this possibility through random assignment of JOBS participants to case managers with smaller (50:1) or higher (100:1) caseloads. While overall participants in Riverside showed the greatest gains among JOBS programs in this and other studies, there were not significant differences in the outcomes of the "more" versus "less intense" case management groups (Riccio et al., 1994). There is now consensus among program planners and researchers that the choice of design and operations of case management must be linked to a program's resources, target population, and community context (Doolittle & Riccio, 1992; Herr & Halpern, 1994; APWA, 1993).

Though rarely studied, informal components such as program philosophy, goals, and service technology clearly constitute the day-to-day workings of case management programs. The one systematic analysis of JOBS programs to look at these issues found evidence suggesting that informal structures and relations do affect programs' effectiveness in achieving participant compliance with the service contract. More successful projects promoted educational and training goals, relied on persuasion and professional treatment to influence participant behavior, and maximized participant choice by providing an option to exit the program (Hasenfeld & Weaver, 1996; Weaver & Hasenfeld, 1997).[16]

In our study of MassJOBS, we found that differences in both formal and informal program operations were clearly linked to the resource bases and connections available to programs in their local communities. In turn, the daily experience of welfare services varied enormously from one site to the next for both providers and participants. For example, one district office offered diverse and flexible training options to participants and was able to refer them to educational programs in English, Spanish, and Russian. A second office, in a different town but the same metropolitan area, had only two training programs to offer clients, and workers there reported several incidents of having to phone local ethnic restaurants for help with translation for prospective clients who spoke no English.

It is ineffective for local offices to have to rely so heavily on case managers' inventiveness to deal with problems that are more predictable, if unique to individual clients. Yet we found few formal interagency relationships (such as formal referral procedures or case conferences) that could help case managers make service linkages. On their part, other service providers in the community were equally unlikely to attempt coordination with welfare offices. Individuals we spoke to in a variety of service agencies uniformly expressed surprise that we should be studying welfare case management, as they did not consider welfare casework to come anywhere near the approach of their own case managers. They also appeared to believe that the welfare office was, at best, irrelevant in providing care to their clients and at worst, a threat, since clients might perceive that any information given the welfare office about the other agency's services could be used to threaten their benefits. As subsequent sections indicate, that perception was both likely and based in real experience.

Working the System: The Tyranny of the Slot

Notwithstanding the claim that case management is a critical JOBS component because of the complex interagency arrangements the program mandates (Gueron et al., 1991; Doolittle & Riccio, 1992), surveys show that case managers actually spend little time contacting and collaborating with other community agencies to connect clients with social services (Hagen & Lurie, 1994a; APWA, 1992). Other demands on their time plus the lack of authority to mandate services work against case managers' referral efforts. In MassJOBS we found that connections with other agencies were haphazard, and workers lacked comprehensive directories of services in their communities. One supervisor noted that her office's only recourse in getting social services was to file an official notification to the Department of Social Services indicating possible child abuse or neglect. Recipients confirmed that caseworkers were not useful in making connections to other services, noting, "You don't even have that conversation with them." This was particularly the case for issues that fail to conform to terms understood within the social welfare system: For example, a woman with chronic fatigue syndrome who had been unable to get Social Security for disability reported being told by case workers, "Well that's not real, . . . what are you coming to us with this problem for?"

What a JOBS program can offer clients may or may not match the background, interests, and needs of incoming participants, but there is nonetheless pressure within the system to fill the existing placement slots. One respondent provided a good illustration of this in the experience of another recipient: "She went in [to the JOBS program] and they said, 'Oh we'll give you this secretarial training . . . program,' and she went into it, and then . . . like four months into the program [she] found that they weren't teaching her much that she didn't already know. . . . She found it wasn't very useful. . . . She has three kids, she can't just take a minimum wage job and feed those kids. . . . They have a certain quota of folks they're supposed to get off of welfare in a certain period of time . . . and a certain number of training programs to fill and so . . . they tried to slot her right into that without any kind of, you know, is this really going to have a future to it. . . ." Several other recipients complained that the training opportunities open to them led only to lower-paying, less-skilled jobs that were "traditional women's work," and, in one local office, the main contracted training programs were indeed for nurse's aides and clerical workers. Noted one recipient, "I wanted to do truck driving and I even told [the welfare office] I had called up . . . one of the biggest truck driving schools, . . . if they just paid for the school, . . . I could do that and . . . I can take my child up to five years old in the truck, you know and I can drive all around the country, and . . . they wouldn't do it, it's not a woman's work . . . And I tried three different offices to see if it's the same answer, it's like the same answer across the board."

Respondents reported having to discover for themselves what their service options were and becoming assertive in finding educational grants and training programs that JOBS would pay for. They found as well that they had to take on much of the work of the system for themselves, and in some cases preferred that to relying on workers they saw as overworked or inept. One described how she ends up monitoring her caseworker: "They write four papers to get one thing done, and I meant that food stamps, I was telling you about going in there and how..[it] took like three months, and that was me calling almost every week, '[caseworker's name], where are those food stamps, you know, are you going to put it in, you didn't send me that letter saying how much you were going to send me, are you going to put it in this month, [caseworker] it's not in this month, I want it, where is it,' you know, and they say, 'it's coming,' well, it's coming is not helping, my child's hungry, I need that $30. . . ."

"You Have to Tell Practically Everything But How Big He Was": Social Images and Social Relations

The negative images of welfare and its recipients seen historically are still apparent in the operations of JOBS programs and in relations between workers and recipients. To be sure, not all programs, and not all relationships, display such negativity. Social images are built into the very framework of the welfare system, however, and can be evident in current procedures regardless of the intent or character of program staff. The emphasis on serving only the truly needy translates, for example, into procedures aimed at detecting recipient fraud and cutting the rolls. Massachusetts AFDC recipients reported to us many instances of being abruptly confronted with having grants cut because of things they were accused of doing. One case in particular illustrates the precariousness of benefits: "This homeless guy gave my address when he got arrested, like out of the blue, right, and the guy from [the housing department] goes down to the police station to check the police logs every now and again, because I'm pretty well known, he saw my address and went, 'that's [her] address' and cut me off of housing [benefits], because I supposedly had somebody living with me, and I had to go through this big thing and they said 'well you have to get a letter from his landlord saying that he doesn't live with you,' I'm like, he's homeless, what am I supposed to do? And then he said 'well you know, under fraud, we can call the welfare people and get you cut off welfare if you don't do this,' and it's like they don't have . . . any communication under positive circumstances, but boy, they'll call welfare up to get, to cut me off. . . ."

Recipients quickly learn and are well aware how images of deservingness and dependency affect them. One noted the response she got to her realization that her job was costing her money: "Because of the raise in my rent and the lowering of my food stamps [following her employment] after about three or four months I was just like, you shouldn't be doing worse here, so I started saving every single receipt of everything I bought . . . and I was losing about twenty to thirty dollars a week, I was having less income by working than by being on welfare . . . once I figured that out I quit my job, there was no, you know . . . who was it, [names a state representative], was that the one that I was crying on the phone to . . . said that the whole ethic of working should have kept me in that job."

Negative stereotypes of welfare recipients come into play particularly when the issue at hand is child support. Describing her intake interview, a recipient depicted a worker and a set of procedures that seemed to have no limit to their intrusiveness: "And so she's asking me these questions, and one of them [was], 'So how many guys were you fooling around with when you were fooling around with the father,' and 'How long did you have a sexual relationship and when did your sexual relationship start and when did it end? . . . You have to tell practically everything but, you know, how big he was. That was one of the questions they didn't ask you. . . ." Another recipient underscored the imagery at work here: "They love to make you feel like, you know, like you're so cheap for sleeping with a guy [when] you don't know what his Social Security number [is], and it's like, 'you tramp,' you know, it's like, well next time I'll take all this information down first. . . ."

Not surprisingly, recipients reported having little trust in the system and little sense of connection with caseworkers. Typifying workers' views of recipients, one noted, "We run into two attitudes, sometimes from the same worker about the same welfare recipient, 'well, I haven't told them about all these services cause they don't really need them right now and . . . they wouldn't understand it, they're not going to remember it till the next time that they'll be here. . . . The other side is, 'well we don't tell them so much that they're going to then cheat,' so you get this . . . attitude of one, they're too stupid or two, they're going to cheat, they're too smart . . . cause then they're going to figure out how to get around the regs [regulations]." In turn, recipients stereotyped workers as inefficient or worse: "They're not working fast, they're just sitting there and then they're grubby looking, and drinking coffee and doughnuts, I mean they're as fat as police officers. . . ."

Our respondents did report having good relationships with some workers, and in particular with the case manager in the local JOBS program, who was variously described as a "saint" and "one of the only sparkles of light down there." This appeared to be related to the caring, personal attitude that person displayed toward recipients, not to any particular function of the case management role. Whether recipients would find a good personal connection was seen as entirely idiosyncratic: "The attitude is that you're lucky that you're getting something and you have no right to complain no matter what is done to you, and there are . . . you know it depends, it really varies social worker to social worker, you have a good social worker they don't treat you that way, but there's no, they don't even see any responsibility to get social workers not to treat people that way. . . ."

Professionals or Bureaucrats: The Tale of the One-Handed Recipient

The casework approach that underlies welfare case management is based on a model of professionalism that may or may not typify actual case management practice. Welfare offices operate with different sets of norms that guide their workers' behavior toward clients (Hasenfeld & Weaver, 1996). Some operate in line with a "bureaucratic rationality approach" emphasizing "rules and procedures, . . . accuracy and efficiency" (Ibid., p. 238). A "professional treatment" approach, in contrast, "recognizes the distinctiveness of the client and augments the facts with professional judgment" (Ibid., p. 239) in making decisions about clients and services.[17] A professional approach to case management would, obviously, be easier to attain in an office adopting the professional treatment approach. Even here, however, professional norms of worker discretion and autonomy conflict with the division of labor, standardized work procedures, paperwork, and administrative time requirements that come with bureaucratic settings.[18]

The challenge for case managers often becomes finding ways to work around the bureaucratic demands of their jobs in order to achieve effective working relations with clients; yet the very requirements of service bureaucracies can vitiate such efforts. One example evident in our research on MassJOBS involved the central welfare office calling for a total reassignment of caseloads in order to safeguard worker objectivity, a prime bureaucratic (and for that matter, professional) value. This reassignment, which had the appropriately symbolic name of an "Alpha Change," was unusual; more commonly, local offices would adjust case assignments periodically to meet overall workload demands. In both cases, continuity of contacts between caseworkers and clients suffered, and one caseworker told us that she rarely saw the same clients through more than one reassessment. While the JOBS program was not directly involved in these reassignments, they compromised the ability of caseworkers to identify appropriate JOBS candidates and provide case managers with adequate information about them.

Caseload demands and continuity issues also limited case managers' ability to detect problems clients were having, though as the last section suggested, clients could also be less than forthcoming with their case manager. One of the more extreme illustrations of how this could affect the ability of a client to move toward employment was reported by a case manager who we found to be very perceptive. She told of getting a phone call from an employer rejecting a client she had known for two years on the grounds that the client was "handicapped." Surprised, the case manager asked what the employer meant and learned for the first time that the client had no left hand.

Attempts to standardize case management procedures may be counterproductive for program goals. One JOBS participant described how the monitoring activities mandated of JOBS case managers were detrimental to her own well-being: Referring to the paperwork required when she went to work, she said, "Yeah, you have to have somebody sign it. And so a lot of people who have jobs, they don't want to have their boss sign it, [and] a lot of bosses don't want to go through the bull of having to . . . fill out all this information every month so they just . . . won't hire you. But if you . . . get your monthly report in late, you're supposed to be working, you're a single parent . . . taking care of a house, God forbid you [don't] send the monthly report in on time, . . . immediately they send you the flyer saying you've been shut off [from benefits]." In another example, all MassJOBS referrals and placements were delegated to MassJOBS workers, even though those who were most ready and able to enter employment might have been better served by a direct job referral by an AFDC staff worker. This was one reason for a major bottleneck in the JOBS program: Of roughly 50,000 mandatory participants in the state at the time of our study, only about 16% were recorded as active in assigned activities.[19]

On the other hand, too much frontline worker discretion can also be counterproductive. At the time of our study of MassJOBS, there was no uniform screening procedure to assess the job-readiness of recipients. This was the case in part because the different constituencies involved in developing such a procedure, including the central office staff, workers, supervisors, union officials, and welfare rights advocacy groups, could not agree on what would be both reliable and fair in such a measure. As a consequence, it was difficult for case managers to be precise in determining which clients were most able to take advantage of employment opportunities, a factor again contributing to their caseload bottleneck.

Other research has found that a professional treatment approach is more likely than one emphasizing "bureaucratic rationality" to promote client compliance with a welfare-to-work plan and to "channel the energies of the staff and participants toward the development of mutual trust, compatibility of objectives, and commitment to success" (Hasenfeld & Weaver, 1996, p. 255). The authors go on to note, however, that such an approach depends on the political economy and civic culture of the program's local community. Given the history of social welfare, it could hardly be otherwise. Structural and procedural changes could enhance the administration, flexibility, specificity, and continuity of case management programs. Given the negative climate undermining the images of both workers and clients, however, it is unlikely that structural changes alone will suffice.

Looking-Glass Case Management

"We all . . . try to do outreach in the welfare office, the most depressing place to do your outreach because everybody's always there feeling downtrodden, you know, if you get them five feet outside the door they're in a better mood than when they're sitting there." This statement, which sounds like that of a trained social worker, was in fact made by a welfare recipient in the JOBS program. It conveys an impression we had frequently when studying JOBS case management: that of looking in a mirror, where the reflection was exactly the opposite of the intended reality.

Instead of an individualized intake and assessment, recipients told us of feeling like they were in a "cattle call," where "you just take a number and sit down"; then, of waiting for hours only to be further dehumanized by the questions with which intake workers confronted them. Care planning consisted of being placed in predetermined slots, with the alternative being to create your own program and opportunities.[20] Case managers reported being able to access social services for participants too late, after things had reached a crisis point; participants reported fears of disclosing needs to caseworkers lest the system do them harm. While case managers spent so much time monitoring participation that they had little opportunity to get to know clients individually, or to get out to stimulate job opportunities, clients also spent a lot of time "monitoring" and "following up" their cases: replacing or refiling forms when the welfare office would lose them, nudging caseworkers to follow up on services, and going through the whole process all over again if they were cut off from benefits.

To be sure, ours was not a random sample of recipients, nor was our study designed as a systematic evaluation of MassJOBS case management. The looking-glass image is intended to convey how case management can break down, and what happens when it does, rather than to represent the typical case. Larger-scale evaluations have, however, identified similar findings (Hagen & Lurie, 1994a, b; APWA, 1992, 1993; Hasenfeld & Weaver, 1996). Under JOBS, case management in some states focused primarily on monitoring client compliance with work participation plans, due to high caseloads and restricted funding. One researcher's observation echoes our looking-glass view: "A focus on case monitoring serves primarily the needs of the agency for information about client status and not client needs for services" (Hagen, 1999, p. 84). States that were aggressive in using benefit terminations when recipients were "out of compliance" with their plans themselves had high rates of errors, with as many as 70% of those disqualified due to inaccuracies in state monitoring and reporting (Hagen, 1999; U.S. General Accounting Office, 1997). Since these plans were devised to emphasize *client* responsibility, we find ourselves again looking in a mirror.

TANF: An End to Welfare, or Welfare As We Have Always Known It?

The Personal Responsibility and Work Opportunity Reconciliation Act of 1996 embodied a fundamental change in social welfare. Abolishing AFDC, JOBS, and related programs, it created in their place the program aptly named *Temporary Assistance for Needy Families* (TANF). TANF departs from AFDC in several respects, but both show continuity with the threads shaping welfare policy in the past. First, TANF completely devolves welfare programs to the states through the mechanism of block grant funding. Unlike the categorical matching of federal and state funds under AFDC, with TANF, each state receives a fixed amount of federal funds based on its prior spending levels for welfare programs. States must not reduce spending on their welfare programs below a certain level, but if they spend only the minimum required for full block grant funding, total state funding could be reduced by one-third in the first six years of TANF operation, compared with what it would have been under AFDC. In addition, eligibility and conditions for receipt of welfare are now completely left up to criteria imposed by states, and there are no federal requirements to serve any specific types of families or individuals. Basically, this "abdicates federal responsibility for needy children by abolishing any entitlement to benefits or services" (Bane, 1997, p. 3, cited in Hagen, 1999, p. 79).

Along with abolishing the federal entitlement to cash assistance, the intent of TANF is to "give a different message to welfare recipient(s): that welfare is not a way of life" (Hagen, 1999, p. 81). The clearest embodiment of this message is the "welfare cliff" (Ibid.) built into TANF, a five-year lifetime limit on receiving assistance through program funds, but there are smaller ledges as well. Recipients must engage in work or work-related programs when the welfare office assesses them as ready to do so, but in any case within two years of starting to receive assistance. The participation rate (proportion of recipients involved in work requirements) mandated for states is higher than that ever expected under JOBS. Work requirements generally entail more hours than under JOBS. Reflecting Congress's preference for a "labor force attachment strategy" rather than a "human capital investment one" (Ibid., p. 80) in reducing dependency, TANF allows fewer forms of educational programs to count as participation requirements, as well as restricting the proportion of recipients in them. Although funding for child care was authorized along with TANF, the program does not guarantee child care for recipients. Recipients who do not comply with work requirements may not just have benefits reduced, but lose them, and not just their own welfare benefits, but those of their entire family. While TANF was the culmination of President Bill Clinton's campaign promise to "end welfare as we know it" (Ibid., p. 79), the images of dependency and the work ethic embedded in the program seem but exaggerated statements of welfare as we have always known it.

Finally, TANF contained the promise of a return to a social service orientation within welfare programs. States are allowed to use funds for social services that are not tied to financial aid eligibility and are thus not subject to time limits. Screenings for possible drug abuse and domestic violence are now mandated as part of intake, the intent being to head off some of the more severe problems keeping clients on welfare by providing intensive case management and referring them to appropriate services. More critically, in order to gain efficiency in providing both income maintenance and employment-related services, states are reorganizing their welfare offices based on the realization that "what they need now are social workers, not clerks" (Lens & Pollack, 1999, p. 74). One approach is to co-locate social services related to job placements with eligibility determination; a second involves "integrated case management" uniting income maintenance and employment services back under the same worker. Although overall the program is very different from the AFDC enacted in 1962, these structures clearly revert to both the form and the intent of that time.

Will going "back to the future" increase the ability of welfare programs to achieve social service goals? Most commentators are skeptical, pointing to several flaws in the plan (Hasenfeld, 2000; Lens & Pollack, 1999; Hagen, 1999). First, the changes ignore the overall context in which welfare is administered, a context based on bureaucratic principles that are incompatible with professional goals. Eligibility determination is similarly incompatible in principle with a social service orientation: The former involves exclusion and an inherently adversarial relation; the latter, inclusion and a working partnership. For example, basing compliance on sanctions compromises the ability of the worker to achieve a relationship with the client based on trust. Moreover, those who are sanctioned tend to be the most difficult cases, precisely those the worker should most want to help. Already foreseeable is a return to the tyranny of the slot, churning, and other victim-blaming procedures typifying welfare as it has been. The fact that TANF does not require program outcome measurement or tracking (just tracking of time on welfare and participation) is telling of the outcomes we can expect: "For less-skilled welfare mothers who avoid the welfare cliff and find employment, the outlook is bleak, especially if measured in terms of reducing or alleviating poverty rather than reducing welfare rolls" (Hagen, 1999, p. 82).

CONCLUSION

Whatever the specifics of welfare programs in the future, it is clear that they will involve case management, and that the role played by case managers will again be transformed to suit the policy requirements of the day. At the same time, case management will continue to reflect the problems that come with the political, economic, organizational, and ideological contexts of welfare programs. Making case management effective thus ultimately requires changing the ways our social structure promotes poverty, the organizational culture of welfare offices, the structure of low-wage work, and the lives of recipients.

No one argues that we have made real progress in achieving the broader goals of welfare through the efforts of the system itself, or through the use of case management. Why, then, have we kept coming back to case management as part of welfare reform? A simple response is that its appeal lies in the low demands it makes for organizational and systemic change; yet case management is not without costs, and within the past quarter century no welfare program could afford to divert its resources ineffectively. Another possibility is that case management serves symbolic purposes important to the system at large, in particular reinforcing negative views of dependency and positive views of work. These images then feed the myths that have always justified welfare as a solution to problems caused by personal pathology rather than by political and economic interests (Hasenfeld, 2000). While persuasive, such explanation fails to account for the specific intent of case management, nor for the agency of both case managers and their clients. Moreover, it cannot explain the success of case management in becoming entrenched in other fields. In the next chapter, we will look across sectors to find some of the reasons for case management's enduring popularity.

NOTES

1. "Not alms but a friend" was the motto of Boston Associated Charities, founded in 1879 (Lubove, 1975, p. 23).
2. This chapter focuses on income support welfare programs, the main site of case management for this sector. The country's major program of this type is Temporary Aid to Needy Families (TANF), which replaced the longstanding Aid to Families with Dependent Children (AFDC) in 1996. Associated programs provide employment, education, and training for recipients, child support enforcement, and benefits for child care, transportation, and other work-related expenses.
3. A(F)DC also persistently endured a negative public image, as shown in nationwide opinion poll findings from the early 1960s through the mid-1980s (Rochefort, 1986, pp. 114–116; Cook & Barrett, 1992). Although this has not necessarily reflected a majority lack of support, compared to other social welfare programs AFDC has been "doubly cursed with less active supporters and more active opponents" (Cook & Barrett, 1992, p. 67).
4. For example, 2% of American children received ADC support in 1940, rising to 4% by 1962 and again doubling to 8% in 1970 (Rochefort, 1986). Economic dislocations, particularly of Southern agricultural workers, were root causes for much of the earlier increases; later growth was fueled as well by the welfare rights movements. For contrasting accounts of these trends, see Axinn and Levin (1997) and Piven and Cloward (1993).
5. As phrased by the Ad Hoc Committee on Public Welfare appointed in 1961 by Secretary of Health, Education, and Welfare Abraham Ribicoff. It is difficult to find a more concrete definition of what these services were in-

tended to be, either in theory or in practice. The "noneconomic services" delivered under AFDC included child care, foster care, and job training and placement, among others. The essence of "prevention and rehabilitation" consisted of personal counseling and social casework delivered by professional social workers. It is also unclear whether the services provided for did anything different from those already offered within state welfare systems, in essence simply giving states a source of increased federal support (Steiner, 1971).

6. Smith and Stone (1988) cite a 1978 study showing more than two-thirds of Title XX expenditures (excluding direct state administrative costs) going to purchased services.

7. That is, standardized assessments of income and assets.

8. Although a BSW credential was accepted by the Council on Social Work Education in 1966, NASW did not admit BSW workers as members until 1970 (Schram & Mandell, 1997), and its membership is still limited to those with a baccalaureate or higher degree.

9. For example, the financial standard used to determine whether a family is in need increased merely 38% from 1970 to 1980, while the Consumer Price Index increased 212% (Handler & Hasenfeld, 1991, pp. 121–122).

10. Take, as an illustration, Chilman's (1992, p. 360) claim that many long-term AFDC families face "a complex of serious family problems with which they need skilled professional help over a period of time." Or the report of findings by the Office of the Inspector General that "learning disabilities and substance abuse were the most widely identified functional impairments for some AFDC recipients, but the study also noted other impairments such as domestic violence, mental and emotional limitations, and the lack of self-esteem, self-motivation, and coping mechanisms" (Hagen & Davis, 1994, p. 69). As the latter also shows, such problems did not exist solely on a discursive level. One survey of AFDC recipients in the mid-1980s found 22% of those under age 45 reporting themselves as disabled, compared to 9% of a comparison group not on AFDC (Adler, 1988). The most common source of disability consisted of back or spine problems, followed by an extensive range of health problems. Similar findings emerged a decade later in a study of JOBS participants in four cities, in which 17% rated their health status fair or poor and 13% related being limited in their ability to work due to health problems (Hagen & Davis, 1994). Moreover, in the latter study, 14% reported that a child had special health problems, and an additional 1% that two children had such problems.

11. For detailed descriptions of programs and their outcomes see Gueron et al., (1991) and Handler and Hasenfeld (1991).

12. Some of the demonstration programs arising at this time also used generalist case managers to provide intensive service intervention, counseling, and coaching to AFDC recipients. This was especially the case for projects targeting participants with multiple needs or heightened vulnerability, such as teenage parents. See Maynard (1993), Herr (1994), and Hamilton et al. (1993) for examples of these case management applications.

13. Mississippi's JOBS program introduced case management into the welfare

arena for the first time in that state and involved a comprehensive, generalist model making the case manager a "client partner" who could advocate for the client and had authority to requisition services and resources
across agency boundaries. Along with this, case managers were located in
the local community action agency and contracted their services with the
state welfare department (Hagen & Lurie, 1994a, p. 6).

14. This work was a Better Government Competition Winner in the 1994 competition sponsored by the Pioneer Institute for Public Policy Research
(Rochefort & Dill, 1994). Dr. David Rochefort (of Northeastern University)
and I identified critical problems in welfare case management in the state
and developed recommendations for change in the system as well as in
practice. We drew on interviews with welfare recipients and with personnel at all levels in various offices of the Massachusetts Department of Public Welfare.

15. See Doolittle and Riccio (1992) for a systematic discussion of these issues
and the intricacies of evaluating these programs.

16. This study analyzed four county programs in GAIN, California's welfare-
to-work program. The authors are unable to draw causal inferences due to
the exploratory nature of the study; neither are they able to control for the
impact of factors such as caseload size or the voluntariness of program participation. They did, however, attempt to rule out other possibly con-
founding variables, such as ethnic differences among the sites. While it is
not possible to ascertain whether the same program characteristics, embedded in a different context with a different client population, would
have the same results, others have similarly emphasized the importance of
the interpersonal connection between case managers and participants (see,
e.g., Hagen & Davis, 1994).

17. The authors also describe a third approach, one of "moral judgment," in
which clients are judged by the moral norms and personal ideologies of
staff.

18. See findings reported by APWA (1992) and Hagen and Lurie (1994a) on the
high proportion of time JOBS case managers spend on paperwork (33–39%
of work time) and in meetings with other staff (9–13.9%).

19. The central welfare office believed the actual number to be somewhat higher because of data entry and monitoring problems. Other major reasons for
the inactive pool were inadequacies in the supply of support services and
placement slots.

20. Some might argue that this type of initiative was precisely what work programs were designed to stimulate. Our respondents were primarily high
school graduates who had joined a support program for welfare recipients;
they were relatively advantaged and took an assertive stance toward their
programs. Others would have fewer skills and less support with which to
pursue alternatives beyond the program slots available to them.

5

Questions Answered
and Unasked*
Themes and Tensions Across Service Sectors

For close to three decades, case management has been a favored instrument of social welfare policy. In examining its history in different service sectors we have had a pinhole view of the changing objectives and prevailing political philosophies of those years. The story of case management would be incomplete without acknowledging its manifestation in an ever-increasing roster of settings. Case management shows every sign of continuing to be the policy mechanism of choice for those who want to rationalize service systems. New versions of the practice are emerging in managed care and private practice, and there has been increased interest in case management in countries where the dissolution of state-dominated service systems has threatened service integration and limited service resources. This chapter looks back across the sectors previously examined as well as at newer applications to ask two questions that, admittedly, can only receive partial answers: Why has case management enjoyed such continued appeal? And, why are there so many different types of structures all carrying the label *case management*? We will see how case management's past, present, and likely future popularity are linked to its role as a bureaucratic tool as well as its grounding in the social structure of our society. We will also see how the diversity of case management forms comes out of the same sources as its appeal: the ability to convey multiple meanings and serve multiple interests.

Examining the diffusion and diversity of case management requires going beyond the administrative and programmatic concerns that have been studied extensively in the course of case management's history. Cutting across program and sector boundaries, these issues address questions of design, efficacy, efficiency, and costs. Some relate to case managers' quali-

fications, training, and organizational role; others, to issues of client targeting and empowerment; yet others to program quality. These are indeed
important questions, and many answers to them can be found in the work
cited in preceding chapters. Our concern here is, however, to treat those
concerns themselves as problematic by asking a different set of questions:
Why do different priorities arise in different sectors at different times?
What features of case management programs have most evaluations ignored? And how have evaluation data on costs, efficacy, and so forth
shaped case management's expansion, or rather failed to do so? Asking
these questions means getting to the crux of case management's legitimacy as a service technology, and in turn to the foundation of its place in service system reform.

CONTINUED SUCCESS, CONTINUAL FAILURE

A steady stream of legislation has steadily extended case management as
a mandated component of human services, over and beyond what we saw
in the previous chapters (see Vourlekis, 1992; Weil & Karls, 1985). The first
legislative flurry was in the 1970s: as part of community-based care for the
elderly under Social Security Amendments, Title XX Social Service Block
Grants, Medicare waivers, Medicaid demonstrations, and Older Americans Act revisions; as a component of NIMH community support programs in the late 1970s; and as a part of mandated services for the
developmentally disabled and for children with special needs.[1] The movement did not abate in the next decades: Case management became part of
requirements in federal funding for services for children in foster care; was
repeatedly expanded in elder services through Older Americans Act revisions; assumed a broader role in Medicaid through OBRA and COBRA provisions;[2] was built into state welfare programs; became part of block grant
services for the homeless as well as substance abuse programs; and was required as part of public funding of community-based care for people with
chronic mental illness. Equal support has come from state and local governments as well as nonprofit foundations. Long-term care and welfare
case management started as state- and local-level demonstration projects,
for example, and the Robert Wood Johnson Foundation was instrumental
in developing case management programs in mental health care, welfare,
and, more recently, care for people with AIDS.

Remarkable as the expansion of case management has been, it is all the
more so given that there has never been unequivocal evidence of its effectiveness at achieving stated goals. The goals of case management are, of
course, as diverse as the populations and services to which it has been ap-

plied. Furthermore, any particular case management program is likely to have multiple goals, given that case management incorporates activities ranging from case finding to care coordination to service advocacy. It is thus not surprising that evaluation research should uncover mixed results when looking at case management outcomes.

The results of such research are more strikingly equivocal than that, however. In sector after sector, evaluation outcomes have been inconsistent, showing at best modest gains and offsetting deficits. In long-term care, case management programs have shown little impact on nursing home or hospital use, while tending to increase, or have little effect on, overall service costs (Capitman, 1986; Kemper, Applebaum, & Harrigan, 1987; Weissert, 1985). For individuals with chronic mental illness, some case management programs have yielded improved client outcomes as well as reduced care costs. Others, however, show no cost savings, or even increases in costs, and insignificant or mixed impacts on client functioning (see reviews in Chamberlain & Rapp, 1991; Rubin, 1992; Solomon, 1992; Mueser, Bond, Drake, & Resnick, 1998; Gorey et al., 1998). Leading evaluation researchers have found welfare-to-work case management able to achieve only some of its many objectives (Gueron, Pauly, & Lougy, 1991; cf. Doolittle & Riccio, 1992).

Commonly complicating such studies, and the interpretation of their findings, are difficulties in measuring costs and outcomes as well as in establishing an adequate comparison group against which to evaluate case-managed clients' costs and outcomes (Weissert, 1985). Thus, it could (and has) been argued that such design flaws have obscured case management benefits (Applebaum & Austin, 1990; Kane, 1988; Rubin, 1992). Yet in the three sectors at hand even the most sophisticated randomized control studies have failed to confirm this view (cf. Brock & Harknett, 1998; Franklin, Solovitz, Mason, Clemons, & Miller, 1987; Gueron et al., 1991; Kemper, 1988; Riccio et al., 1994). Responding to such mixed or negative results, case management researchers and program designers initially emphasize improving program and study designs, better client targeting, fine-tuning of program components and objectives, or more sensitive outcome measures. Later studies making those improvements have continued to show equivocal results, leading to calls for more realistic and focused expectations of case management as well as to outright skepticism about its utility overall (see, for example, Applebaum & Austin, 1990; Austin, 1990; Doolittle & Riccio, 1992; Franklin, 1988; Kane, 1988; Moore, 1992; Weissert, 1985).

Clearly, the reasons for case management's initial popularity and continued expansion do not lie in its demonstrated efficacy or cost-effectiveness. What, then, are the reasons for case management's success? Most analysts draw on a common account emphasizing the importance of service coordination as a policy trend. In this account, the explosion of service systems in the 1960s led to fragmentation, duplication, inefficiency, and confusion in their organization. Case management, the story continues, emerged first as a way of removing bureaucratic hurdles to service access for individuals with multiple, complex service needs. As funding for service programs grew more scarce throughout the 1980s and to the present, the managerial side of case management came forward (see Austin, 1990; Moore, 1992; Vourlekis, 1992; Weil & Karls, 1985). In a more critical vein, analysts sometimes continue to note that one reason for case management's popularity is that it does not seek fundamental structural change, nor does it ask much of provider agencies; case management "does not significantly alter the relationship and the distribution of resources among providers in local delivery systems" (Austin, 1990, p. 398). Indeed, promoting case management allows policymakers and program planners to make a reform effort while diverting attention (including their own) from a situation of inadequate resources (Austin, 1990; Moore, 1992).

This story is not so much wrong as incomplete. It can discuss the equivocal outcomes of case management programs only as technical failures and therefore neglects to explain the persistence of case management despite them. Furthermore, it does not assess how there can be consensus among many groups and sectors that this particular practice is good although there has never been an exact definition—or consensus—regarding what that practice is. The standard account also does not give reasons for the variability in case management practice within and between service sectors, nor does it assess why consensus about the structure of case management has been so elusive.

THE ROOTS OF SUCCESS

Looking across long-term care, mental health, and welfare, we can identify three sets of factors propelling case management despite its vagueness and frailties. The first derives precisely from the fact that case management programs have themselves been part of broader policy sweeps. The initial explosion of case management in the 1970s occurred as part of efforts at all governmental levels to centralize and coordinate the vast array of public assistance programs created in the prior decade. Including programs such as community action and area health planning agencies as well as case management, the development of coordinating mechanisms was a rationalizing strategy intended to reform and improve extant services rather than implement new ones (Scott, 1991). In mental health, long-term care, and other domains, the mounting of case management also accompanied policy emphases on deinstitutionalization and the creation of community-based care systems, themselves dependent on coordinating mechanisms (Rochefort, 1986; Estes, 1979).

Reflecting the social and fiscal conservatism of the late 1970s and 1980s, coordination increasingly encompassed goals of cost-effectiveness as well. While political interest in competition and capitation foundered in the actual implementation and dissemination of programs (the initially turgid growth of HMOs being a prime example), case management became "the philosopher's stone of cost containment" because of the perception that it could maximize the use of service resources (Spitz & Abramson, 1987). More recently, the political emphasis on service system rationalization has been expressed through policies of privatization and quality assurance, trends again seen in case management practice in long-term care, mental health, and welfare (Donahue, 1989; Raiff & Shore, 1993). Even where regulation offered funding inducements to adopt case management, then, the political promotion of case management has not occurred sui generis, but rather as part of more general policy themes and programmatic thrusts propelling it along.

In each service sector it is possible to identify a constituency for the funding of case management programs or an interest group actively pressing for their endowment. These, then, represent a second factor propelling case management's momentum. In long-term care, these players came from public and nonprofit agencies already providing services and engaged in coordinating activities under the Older Americans Act. In mental health and welfare, service professionals and their associations formed additional constituencies.

For nursing and social work in particular, case management formed part of "professional projects," the process of building infrastructures, networks, constituencies, superstructures to support the enterprise of the profession (Larson, 1977; Bower, 1992; Greene, 1992). Professional groups had a stake in the development of case management because it provided a new opportunity for professional advancement for their membership and because it countermanded the de-skilling of workers prevalent in all service sectors from the late 1970s on. Professionals also contributed to the spread of case management through the development of knowledge bases about client needs, service pathways, assessment and record systems, and so forth. These then appeared to represent best-practice techniques and facilitated the application of case management to new settings lured by the appeal of a new practice appearing to enjoy both professional and bureaucratic support (Raiff & Shore, 1993; cf. Scott, 1991).

A third factor in case management's spread involves its utility for service agencies. The timing of case management's first flourishing generally coincides with a period of high turbulence in the environments surrounding human service organizations. In the case of the early long-term care demonstrations, the sources of this turbulence included the new federalism promoted by President Nixon as well as the block grants consolidating formerly categorical funds. Community mental health and welfare programs were even more directly assailed by reduced federal appropriations and block granting in the second half of the 1970s (Estes, 1979; Rochefort, 1986).

These events placed local agencies at risk by removing more direct administrative and funding connections to federal sources and by making allocation decisions subject both to new players and to interagency competition for a stake in each year's state budget (Estes, 1979). The economic malaise of the time—rampant inflation combined with recession—limited states' purchasing power and revenue yields, intensifying the fiscal pressures on both public and nonprofit providers (Honnard, 1985).

At the same time, service sectors were undergoing revolutionary changes in organization and philosophy. Both long-term care and mental health were attempting to shift from a centralized institutional base to a more complex, decentralized structure of services in the community (Rochefort, 1986). Welfare services, in contrast, were becoming more centralized under state auspices, but with increased need for community connections supporting employment and training programs. In each sector, these changes required concomitant shifts in staffing patterns, roles, functions, knowledge and skill bases, as well as interagency relationships (Honnard, 1985).

More general trends have also been responsible for the need of human welfare programs for a protean technology, one that can change form without losing other instrumental properties. It should be recalled that most social welfare arenas (and specifically, long-term care, primary care, mental health, and income assistance programs) have witnessed within one generation the evolution and devolution of public control. The contraction of a formerly unassailable nonprofit sector and the ascendance of the corporation have further intensified the environmental turbulence encountered by those programs, requiring quick strategic adaptation as well as predictable sources of legitimization.

While public policy has provided the impetus and direction for these transformations, it did not designate the mechanisms through which to achieve them. Under these circumstances, human service organizations have needed ways to monitor connections with their environments, to sense the pulse of funding sources as well as to feel out the competition. They further needed flexibility in their service provision. Whatever mechanisms they chose would have to be introduced at minimal cost, monetarily as well as in terms of fit with standing procedures. It would also have to be recognizable to payers and other agencies as a useful and legitimate service component. Case management offered all these advantages, simultaneously connecting service agencies with funding streams, clientele, and other providers. The pulls of environmental turbulence thus appear at least as important to case management's success as the pushes of professional interests and policy mandates.

THE ROOTS OF DIVERSITY

Looking again at these policy, professional, and environmental factors can also help us understand how it is possible to view the expansion of case management as an ongoing natural experiment in which the experimental variable has kept changing regardless of, or even despite, equivocal feedback on its results. Case management has been resistant to standardization, in form or even in definition. Definitions show a disarming vagueness about its essential elements: "Case management is essentially a problem-solving function designed to ensure continuity of services and to overcome systems rigidity, fragmented services, misutilization of certain facilities and inaccessibility" (JCAH, 1976, cited in Levine & Fleming, 1986, p. 7); or, "a set of logical steps and a process of interaction within a service network which assure that a client receives needed services in a supportive, effective, efficient, and cost effective manner" (Weil & Karls, 1985:2); or, "an intervention using a human service professional . . . to arrange and monitor an optimum package of . . . services" (Applebaum & Austin, 1990, p. 5).

Similarly, there is little conclusive evidence about which case management features or model produces the best outcomes. Even the most systematic, experimental efforts to assess the relative advantages of design options yield few outcome differences, and those few are as likely to disappoint as validate the advocates of different approaches (see, for example, Doolittle & Riccio, 1992; Gorey et al., 1998; Gueron et al., 1991; Kemper, 1988; Mueser et al., 1998; Riccio et al., 1994). Again, it clearly is not demonstrated efficacy or efficiency that has promoted the development of so many permutations, or of particular variations on the theme.

When viewed historically, the ambiguity and variability of case management emerge as both intentional and unintentional consequences of social policy, professional dynamics, and organizational strategies. In no sector has the legislation authorizing case management specified its substance, activities, mechanisms, or objectives at an operational level (Spitz & Abramson, 1987). Avoiding issues of policy implementation while adopting legislation has been a modus operandi long favored by Congress and clearly evident in the creation of the programs that fostered case management. Acting as a circuit breaker to avoid an overload of public demand for welfare initiatives from the Great Society era onward, such legislation was popular on many fronts: among politicians, for facilitating legislative action and thus enhancing their legitimacy; among state and local agencies, for funding new programs that could achieve policy objectives simply by being created (Binstock & Levin, 1976). What the legislation initially promoting case management fostered, then, was a "process without substance" (Spitz & Abramson, 1987, p. 364)—or rather, a process with substance defined at the programmatic level, where professional and organizational interests could prevail.

Although groups of professionals have networked through meetings, associations, and the literature to promote case management,[3] they have not achieved a uniform vision of what case management is or should be. This is particularly apparent when surveying the early literature on case management in any given sector, which debates (with predictability but without resolution) the comparative value of alternative case management designs. Professional groups have also been much divided over questions of case managers' qualifications and standards for the role (Raiff & Shore, 1993). Such discussions grew particularly combative in mental health and social welfare, as the dominant professions (psychiatry and social work, respectively) found their roles challenged by paraprofessionals as part of broader battles over the division of labor in the field (Scott & Backman, 1990; see also Deitchman, 1980; Friday, 1986; Lamb, 1980; Rapp & Chamberlain, 1985; Pecora & Austin, 1983; Wyers, 1980). Moreover, there has been increased acceptance of the idea that case management is multidisciplinary in nature and thus requires the perspectives and involvement of a variety of professionals. This has "neutralized the claim . . . to monopoly" (Raiff & Shore, 1993, pp. 10, 12) over case management standards or practice by any one profession and has promoted the development of multidisciplinary teams, which divert issues of professional turf from a collective level to that of frontline service delivery.

At the organizational level, the ambiguity attached to the definition of case management meant that agencies could adjust case management features to whatever they needed and were able to mount at a given time. Recall the commentary likening mental health case management to "a Rorschach test" onto which "an individual, an agency, or a community will project . . . its own particular solution to the problems it faces in providing community-based care for the chronic mentally ill" (Schwartz, Goldman, & Churgin, 1982, p. 1006). Certainly, particular types and models of case management have been imitated, but what agencies copied more was what the term *case management* subsumed: a set of ideals, processes, and relationships rather than structures and positions. In short, the concept itself has become institutionalized.

Thus far we have pointed to the momentum of social policy, the entrepreneurial actions of professionals, and organizational needs of service providers as sources of both case management's entrenchment and its variability. Yet, policy trends, professional dynamics, and organizational strategies have also favored other, less permanent forms of service technology. To understand why the concept of case management has such enduring appeal, we need to look more closely at what it includes—and what it leaves out.

DOMINANT CULTURAL SYMBOLS

A leading analyst of human service organizations notes that the growth and survival of such organizations "depends less on the technical proficiency of their work and more on their conformity with dominant cultural symbols and beliefs systems" that form an "institutional environment" (Hasenfeld, 1992, p. 10). This conformity is also a crucial factor for choices made about service technologies like case management: "Technologies ascend in importance as they gain greater legitimacy in the institutional environment. They do so through their demonstrated capacity to reinforce important values and norms" (Ibid., p. 12; see also Albrecht & Peters, 1995). Since, as we have seen, it is not the demonstrated technical proficiency of case management that led to its ascendance within different service sectors, we need to ask what "dominant cultural symbols" and "values and norms" it reinforces. To some extent, we have done this in the chapter on each sector, and subsequently review some of the specific values attached to different case management applications. To begin with, however, we need to pull back and assess case management's symbolic importance on a broader level.

First, case management is a bureaucratic mechanism and as such reproduces and communicates the symbolic order of service bureaucracies. Even when not situated in a bureaucratic agency, case management serves bureaucratic purposes in that it attempts to compress distinct individual situations into the basis for routinized official decisions (see Friedland & Alford, 1991). Procedures of assessment, care planning, and service connections thus rationalize the life worlds of clients, converting their narratives to categories of *need* and *entitlement* (Dill, 1993). The very focus on the individual as the locus of the problem reflects broader forces in the rationalization of American social bureaucracies since the Progressive era.

At the institutional level (if not necessarily that of service organizations), case management elaborates the attempts of the state to rationalize and regulate human activity. Its location at the interface between lay and official realms places it at "a crucial point of articulation wherein ... discrepancies of connection and communication are most likely to be evident," a site where are revealed "the coercion and fragility of structures of power" (Handelman & Leyton, 1978, p. 6). By representing the client to the bureaucracy, case management seeks to provide protection from those elements of coercion; hence, its advocacy functions. By representing the bureaucracy to the client, case management equally protects bureaucratic structures from their fragility: their inability to tolerate "conflicting claims over the substantive ends toward which bureaucratic rationality is directed or demands for popular participation in them" (Friedland & Alford, 1991, p. 249). Case management, in short, contains exceptionalism, having the ability to offer as well as to withhold it.

This mediating role represents, in miniature, a system of checks and balances to the power of public bureaucracy. It reflects particular American notions: a penchant for restraint of centralized authority as well as a "negative" concept of freedom—"freedom *from*" institutional powers (Friedland & Alford, 1991, p. 246). Case management has become an essential bureaucratic apparatus in large part because public policy has made services available along categorical lines defined by certain attributes of clients, such as their age, resources, or physical or mental condition. This again reflects broader cultural predilections: a focus on individual sources of problems rather than social structural ones, for example, or the conceptual isolation of *medical* from *social* needs. These categories denote exclusion as well as inclusion, and the organization of service sectors along categorical lines has excluded attention to those whose needs are not so neatly typified (Scott, 1991; cf. Herzfeld, 1992). The policy solution has been to emphasize coordination across sectors as an objective of service systems (Estes, 1979). Since the problem has been defined as one of accommodating individual variation, case management provides a culturally suitable means toward that end.

Case management is not purely a bureaucratic mechanism, however. The fact that case managers act as "the human link" between the client and the system (Baker & Weiss, 1984, p. 925) also means that their role combines social relations like those of primary group members with those of bureaucratic functionaries (Dill, 1987). Like kin, case managers take on a diffuse responsibility for client welfare, have extensive one-to-one contact with clients, focus on issues of daily functioning, and make long-term (programmatic) commitments. This, then, confronts the rationalizing logic of bureaucracy with familial commitments to community and loyalty. What happens as a result of mixing these contradictory elements depends largely on the symbolic order of particular service sectors.

THE CULTURE OF SERVICE SECTORS

American culture has shaped particular service sectors through the ways social problems and populations are categorized and typified. The constructs pertinent here include assumptions, beliefs, and values held about clients, the origins of social problems, and the structures and expertise appropriate to the solution of those problems. Thus, case management in long-term care drew from (and in turn reinforced) a particular social construction that defined the problems of older people as amenable to service intervention and justified such intervention as an entitlement owing to the "deservingness" of the elderly (Estes, 1979; see also Rochefort, 1986). These constructs had been institutionalized through Older Americans Act provisions and the growth of the aging enterprise well in advance of the advent of case management structures. Similarly, the promotion of case management in mental health fit with the perceived benefits of community integration of the mentally ill, the theorized social etiology of mental problems, and a growing distrust of orthodox psychiatry as well as bureaucratic structures within the sector at large (Rochefort, 1986). In welfare, case management developed in a context centered on the contract between citizen and society and on negative perceptions of dependency.

The policy and service entrepreneurs who deployed case management in each sector communicated these wider meanings, reinforcing the social constructions legitimating their sectors' forms and approaches. At the same time, those entrepreneurs were politicizing the tensions introduced into sectors by the contradictory logics and values accruing to case management. In both long-term care and mental health, the original framing of case management was as a reform effort, an attempt to provide the human link that would allow a degree of particularism and familistic concern to enter bureaucratic service provision. In welfare, arguably the most politicized of service sectors, case management offered a mechanism acceptable both to those favoring the individualized and trusting relations of social services and to those seeking greater bureaucratic efficiencies.

The mixture of different values and social meanings within case management is also evident in the issues that become of primary concern in the shaping of programs in particular service sectors. One of the main design debates in long-term care case management has centered on the degree of resource control that needs to be accorded case managers. On one side is the brokerage model, in which case managers act as referral agents and advocates but cannot directly allocate services or funds; on the other, in service management or managed care models, case managers have complete control over pooled funding sources and service provision (Applebaum & Austin, 1990). Concern about the relative effectiveness and cost containment potential of these different designs was sufficient to justify a major federal demonstration project, the Channeling experiment (Carcagno & Kemper, 1988). The correlations of brokerage with informal (familial) caregiving, on the one hand, and of service management or managed care with bureaucratic rationalization, on the other, are clearly not accidental.

The situation in mental health has been more complex and illustrates how groups contend for dominance within service sectors by attempting to politicize competing values. Countering the medical model of mental illness embedded in orthodox psychiatry and institutional care, community mental health promoters invoked public health idioms of etiology and treatment (Rochefort, 1986). Some psychiatrists, while supporting these models and the concept of community-based care, nonetheless continued to argue the importance of combining the case manager role with that of clinician, citing the therapeutic importance of the professional-client relationship (Lamb, 1980; Dietchman, 1980). More recently, consumer groups have countered both bureaucratic and professional rationalities by asserting the primacy of values based on the concepts of popular participation and empowerment. The current shape of much of mental health case management—an interdisciplinary team approach incorporating environmental context assessment as well as client goals—reflects a symbolic as well as material compromise among these competing values, and among the interests advancing them (Raiff & Shore, 1993).

The uneasy fit of a social service orientation within the welfare bureaucracy has been evident throughout case management's deployment in that sector. Images of the moral worth of clients inherent in a social service approach are hard to sustain in a system based on excluding all but the "truly needy." We saw in Chapter 4 how the use of bureaucratic measures to ensure impartiality can confound attempts by case managers to develop ongoing relationships with clients. The emphasis on monitoring and sanctioning, again bureaucratic elements, too readily work against building trusting, change-producing relations (Hasenfeld, 2000). Debates within the field have centered precisely on elements of bureaucratic structure: the criteria and standards for case managers; whether to merge or separate income eligibility with case management work; the intensity of case management, translated as caseload size. Only slightly below the surface, however, are the broader questions of values driven by images of worth, dependency, and work.

CULTURE AND DIFFERENCES IN PRACTICE

So far we have examined the meanings and values embedded in case management when assessed at the level of service sectors. We should not expect to find the same symbolic elements reproduced throughout a given set of case management programs, however. *Culture* is neither so homogeneous nor so determinative, but rather constitutes a "tool kit of symbols, stories, rituals and world-views, which people may use in varying configurations to solve different kind of problems" (Swidler, 1986, p. 273). The diverse values attached to case management have made it a cultural tool of powerful ambiguity, and the meanings it expresses therefore vary both across and within sectors as well as through time.

Case management in one organization will differ from that in another depending on the different values and ideologies that guide their missions and operations and that are available to actors establishing the organization's material and social relations. Beliefs about what is good for clients (practice ideologies) and choices of service technologies tend to operate in a loop of mutual feedback, creating a self-referential system of assumptions that operates at a taken-for-granted level. Views of welfare clients as "morally deficient," for example, will justify very different practices from those seeing clients as lacking "human capital" (Hasenfeld & Weaver, 1996, p. 239). Case management in any particular organization may also differ from that in another area because of aspects of the local context related to the presence of politicizing actors (such as community elites) and wider tensions, such as those based in racial or labor relations.

The configuration of symbolic elements attached to case management may also have different uses at different levels within the system; thus, what "works" at the level of social policy may look very different at the level of frontline practice. This type of disconnect between policy and practice is typical of boundary-spanning positions and commonly found in social welfare fields. It enables the production of situations in which social policy can appear to achieve its objectives, all the while displacing value conflicts to the frontline worker (Handler & Hasenfeld, 1991; Horowitz, 1995).

While the contradictory values embedded in case management are particularly evident in the field of welfare, value conflicts are almost certainly responsible for part of the role strain reported for workers in various service sectors (Applebaum & Austin, 1990; Doolittle & Riccio, 1992; Intagliata & Baker, 1983; Levine & Fleming, 1986; Weil, 1985b; see also Kane, Penrod, & Kivnick, 1994). The connections with diverse meanings and logics lead to different and potentially contradictory role requirements for case managers, as well as a variety of constituencies with interests in their work. Being an advocate in a relationship with a client may not mesh well with acting as a gatekeeper for system resources, to take one obvious example. Case managers must not only merge these role sets, they must translate among them, entering the diverse discourses they embody and communicating with role partners in ways that differ substantively and philosophically (Dill, 1990).

Differences in practice among case managers emerge, then, from the value constellations surrounding their work as well as from their individual skills and preferences. This may explain research findings that the ways in which case managers categorize and perceive client needs are closely linked to what they can do with and for the client (Phillips, Kemper, & Ap-

plebaum, 1988; Chamberlain & Rapp, 1991). While organizational structures provide the constraints and opportunities for individual action, individuals work strategically within and against those bounds, manipulating
ambiguities and contradictions in defining the meaning of their work. For
example, social workers acting as mental health case managers commonly "drift" toward counseling, in line with the higher status of a therapeutic role within their profession (Curry, 1980, Johnson & Rubin, 1983). On
the other hand, a demonstration mental health project serving children and
adolescents found the amount of case management to be inversely related
to the severity of the child's problems, but positively associated to the overall level and amount of non-case management services received. These
outcomes suggest the administrative pressures on case managers to be
agents of cost and service control (Hamner & Bryant, 1997), pressures observed for all systems under managed care. The sensitivity of case management to organizational and professional climates has also been found
in services for people with AIDS, especially within hospitals, where a direct care orientation prevails (Piette, Fleishman, Mor, & Dill, 1990; see also
Austin, 1990; and Fiorentine & Grusky, 1990).

OUTSIDE THE CULTURAL FRAME:
THE INVISIBLE WOMAN

So far we have examined case management's popularity and variability by
teasing out its cultural meanings and how they are expressed in particular
service sectors and programs. Case management has become an institutionalized cultural practice connoting core symbolic constructs attached to
service systems. These include constructs at many levels: those representing systems' or programmatic attributes and objectives (e.g., fragmentation, coordination, continuity of care, deinstitutionalization, community-
based care, bureaucratic standards), those that define the locus of problems
and the nature of service dynamics (individual need, caregiving, assessment, care planning), and those typifying particular categories of people
(the deserving elderly or the welfare mother). These constructs constitute
the taken-for-granted culture of service systems and provide the rhetoric
and rationale for the development of case management. In turn, case management reinforces its symbolic building blocks, adding to them the
knowledge base of frontline practice as well as the imprimatur of legislative, organizational, and professional authority.

But equally important to case management's rise, spread, and ultimate
fate are symbolic elements that are excluded from this construction. Defining case management as a service technology (whether bureaucratic or
professional) leaves opaque the social and material relations constituting

case management practice. Personal attributes of clients are relevant in this discourse only insofar as they are believed to affect program outcomes. Personal attributes of case managers are relevant only insofar as they might explain practice variations. In both cases, the attributes considered within practice and evaluation literature tend to be those bearing direct reference to the system itself: for example, how many times a client has been a client, or the types of services received; or how long a case manager has worked within the system or in the same position.

A central aspect of case management left out of this picture is the fact that it is work generally done by women on behalf of female clients. It is difficult to provide precise statements about the extent to which females outnumber males as case managers, since studies of case management programs seldom report the sex of their staff.[4] In and of itself, this is a meaningful omission, denoting the bureaucratic assumption that persons are separable from offices and hence that workers are individuals only in the abstract (Friedland & Alford, 1991). It further mirrors the invisibility often attached to caregiving and other areas of "women's work," which this culture constructs as within a domain of private rather than public concern (Abel, 1991; Rodeheaver, 1987). Where case management is done primarily by social workers, nurses, or so-called pink collar paraprofessionals, the gender imbalance may be presumed to reflect that of those occupations. The gender balance of workers is likely to be reversed only when physicians have been case managers (e.g., Medicaid primary care and some mental health programs) and in early case management efforts for people with AIDS, largely mounted by community-based advocacy groups of gay men (Mor, Fleishman, Allen, & Piette, 1994).

The clientele of case management programs are also disproportionately women: in long-term care, by virtue of their greater longevity and higher levels of functional dependency than men; in welfare because the focus has been on AFDC recipients. There is a gender loading even in mental health, perhaps related to the greater overall tendency of women to be care seekers (Nathanson, 1977). Although reports on case management programs are more likely to document the sex of clients than that of staff, this information forms a demographic background used mainly as evidence of the representativeness of the client sample compared to an appropriate population. It is not ascribed substantive or theoretical significance.

Yet the fact that case management often boils down to women caring for women is significant. First, such case management programs reproduce the organization of gender within the human services (Hasenfeld, 1992). Although in some times and sectors, social work and nursing have been able to use case management strategically to enhance the professionalism of their fields, in other areas (particularly mental health and public civil service systems) the trend has been toward de-skilling their work with the use of paraprofessionals (Austin, 1990). Such upward occupational mobility as case management has provided has come with a glass ceiling: Case managers may aspire to become case management supervisors, but there is no straight line beyond that to positions of higher authority. Following trends in other human service fields, moreover, we would expect women to be underrepresented in those administrative jobs, paid less than men in comparable positions, and receiving lower wages and less status than workers in male-dominated occupations (Hasenfeld, 1992).

A second area of significance arises from the contradictions of family and bureaucratic logic built into the concept of case management. Like women's domestic and caregiving labor, case management requires working within family systems, negotiating and networking, and assembling some coherent order out of an array of often incongruous pieces (Rodeheaver, 1987). Both its means and its ends may differ from those dictated by bureaucratic procedures; the "caring" quality of relationships with clients and the "emotion work" case managers perform, for example, do not fit well with standardized outcome measures and performance assessments (McAuley, Teaster, & Safewright, 1999). The less they end up being counted, the less the familistic sides of case management "count" in programmatic or policy terms (cf. Diamond, 1986). They still count for case managers, however, who may adapt by trying to "game" more rigid bureaucratic requirements or suffer role strain when such efforts fail (McAuley, Teaster, & Safewright, 1999).

Finally, the insignificance attached to client gender in studies of case management programs keeps veiled the structural sources of the problems those programs are supposed to address. Again elaborating the institutional logic of service bureaucracies, the problem is defined and located at the connection of the individual with the service provider. Broader issues of the systematic economic disadvantages faced by women throughout the life course simply do not fit in this picture.

Although there is even less indication in the case management literature of similar class or ethnic and racial imbalances among case management staff, those are also issues worth pursuing. In terms of the composition of clientele, by one estimate people of color now constitute almost 40% of the clients of social service systems (Raiff & Shore, 1993). In sectors where case management is a function of public services, clients are likely to come disproportionately from lower-class and/or ethnic minority backgrounds. At work to produce these imbalances are interlinked cultural and structural factors: discrimination, the stresses of immigration and acculturation, and the lack of culturally accessible and acceptable care. These complicate both service needs and the work of case managers in multiple ways (Raiff & Shore, 1993). Although there has been increased attention to "cultural competency" and sensitivity as components of case management practice

(Raiff & Shore, 1993, pp. 65–77), this still defines the problem as one of re-tooling the technology to match the culture of the client. Broader structural implications are again left for a different venue.

THE PAST AS PROLOGUE

By combining the analysis of case management's cultural meanings with that of its material and social institutions, we can now claim a better understanding of both its endurance and its variability, which can, in turn, help us assess ongoing developments and newer applications of case management practice. The "stock of culturally available legitimating 'accounts'" (DiMaggio & Powell, 1991, p. 21) that have justified case management historically drew heavily from the assumptions and values buttressing state bureaucracies, in general, and human service sectors, in particular. The early incentives for adopting case management approaches relate to the instability and turbulence experienced by those sectors, conditions when "successful collective action often depends upon defining and elaborating widely accepted rules of the game" (DiMaggio & Powell, 1991, p. 30). The efficacy of those rules is somewhat beside the point, although actors can profit in many ways from adopting accepted symbolic practices. Case management provided a symbolic currency in which organizations could invest at low cost, a set of repeatable routines which they could easily maintain and transmit (cf. Zucker, 1991), and dividends of legitimacy and (at least potentially) enhanced control over service resources.

It has therefore not been necessary for organizations, sectors, or professions to develop a common operational definition of case management, nor to demonstrate its efficacy, for it to become one of the rules of the game. Moreover, case management continued to be viewed as a rational solution to systemic woes because it could be embedded in different programmatic contexts, themselves legitimized by specific rationales and ideologies. This flexibility (which would be precluded by too common or technical a definition) derives from the diverse institutional principles and values built into the concept of case management and the role of case manager: the commitment to long-term, individualized care, like that provided by family members; the bureaucratic concern with both entitlement and efficiency; the use of techniques based in the cognitive frameworks of the helping professions. The form and process of case management in particular sectors and settings have varied with the prevalent balance among these values and the presence of factions interested in politicizing them.

Current developments in case management continue to expand both the areas to which it is applied and the trends and values it incorporates. The array of sites and populations serviced by case management now includes primary care physicians' offices, acute care hospitals, regional health care systems, homeless individuals, high-risk pregnant women, substance abuse treatment programs, HIV risk reduction projects, lifetime care programs for persons with spinal cord injury, school-based services for teenage parents, and military family advocacy units (Ciosci & Goodman, 1994; Cohen & Cesta, 1994; Czerenda & Best, 1994; Davis, 1992; Gemmill, Kennedy, Larison, Mollerstrom, & Brubeck, 1992; Hurley & Fennell, 1990; Netting, Warrick, Christianson, & Williams, 1994; Siegal, 1994; White, Gundrum, Shearer, & Simmons, 1994).

The most notable recent applications of case management are not in new sectors, however, but by new providers. Beginning in the 1980s, case management became a core technology of managed health and mental health care, in traditional HMO settings, in Social/HMOs serving older clients, and in both self-insured and third-party insurance programs. Most major insurance companies now operate with in-house or contracted case management components. Initially focused primarily on high-cost patients, the objectives of managed care case management have since broadened to wider attempts to ration utilization and contain costs incurred by subscribers as a whole (Austin, 1990; Austin & O'Connor, 1989; Hurley & Fennell, 1990; Vourlekis, 1992).

Present trends in health and social services indicate continued reliance on case management programs, but in service contexts increasingly based on prospective, consolidated, capped, and/or capitated funding structures. Placing providers at financial risk reintroduces market forces to sectors formerly relatively shielded from them and promotes more emphasis on gatekeeping and service-rationing activities within case management programs. It further requires that case managers augment their skills in fiscal management and monitoring of case loads (Austin, 1990).

Given the more standardized nature of these procedures, there is likely to be increased reliance on computerized information systems and other technical devices. At some levels, this may promote increased homogeneity in case management structures and operations. At present, however, individual case management programs in welfare, mental health, and other fields are creating their own computer record systems guided as much by local programmatic needs (and in some cases, the desire to market the system they develop) as by technical criteria. It is likely that the multiple interests advanced by case management will thus continue to provide a source of variegation even for more systematic operations.

A related and noteworthy innovation is that of private practice case management. Provided mainly by social workers, fee-for-service case management providing care coordination and monitoring has become a popular resource for elders and their families as well as parents with mentally disabled children (Vourlekis, 1992). This has become a sufficiently large enterprise to warrant the development of professional associations certifying and representing private care managers, such as the Individual Case Management Association, the Commission for Case Manager Certification, and the National Association of Geriatric Care Managers. Allied in a market orientation, if not in service goals or populations, are case management in Employee Assistance Programs and that performed by private firms for public agencies, such as welfare and child welfare departments (Doolittle & Riccio, 1992; Hegar, 1992; N. Miller, 1992). Predictably, case management has also entered the private sector in the form of virtual reality: the "Case Management Resource Guide" enables Web users to search a directory of "over 110,000 healthcare services, facilities, businesses and organizations" providing home care, long-term care, subacute care, psychiatric services, medical products, and more (Dorland Healthcare Information, 1999, www.cmrg.com).

As this discussion conveys, a two-class system of case management is becoming increasingly apparent. On one side are public programs: subject to ever-tightening fiscal constraints, they are decreasing the service resources available to case managers even as they remove the educational requirements for those positions, in short de-skilling them. Market-driven policies have also vitiated the nonprofit service sectors, which originated case management, forcing remaining agencies to act and look like the private sector, or to face absorption into it (Estes, Swan, & Associates, 1993). In contrast, the private sector is providing a new niche for workers with professional backgrounds. One national survey found that over one-third of private case management providers employed only MSWs and close to two-thirds had at least one MSW case manager. The offerings of these agencies included services predictable for an upper middle class market: estate management (reported by 10.3%), financial counseling (26.5%), psychotherapy (34.2%), and financial assessment (77.8%; Secord 1987, reported in Austin, 1990).

As case management becomes more and more a commodity or tool of the marketplace, the values of business, and more broadly of capitalism, join those historically present as unquestioned objectives (Padgett, 1998). Expansion and profit, standardization and predictability, centralized control and efficiency: These fit readily with some of the bureaucratic incentives of case management programs, but uneasily with desires to personalize the client's connection with service systems. Frontline case managers are again left with the job of sorting out the relative "moral claims" of their own agencies, clients, corporate providers, or payers, and society at large (Ibid., p. 8).

CASE MANAGEMENT AND THE WELFARE
MIX: INTERNATIONAL PERSPECTIVES

Since the mid-1980s, case management has spread internationally, finding a home in countries as diverse as Sweden, France, and Australia, and in services for groups ranging from the elderly, mentally ill, and disabled adults to children of drug addicts and survivors of incest. These developments arose in a context marked by common political and economic trends. Economic stringency was in force worldwide, and the tenor of politics shifted to the right. National governments were seeking to devolve responsibility for service systems to more local-level authorities. In line with this was an emphasis on local-level service coordination and consolidation. Policy changes not only permitted but favored the provision of services by private and voluntary organizations, encouraging a more competitive, market-driven orientation in health and social welfare. In this pluralistic "welfare mix" the roles of purchaser and provider now divided, and historical splits widened between medical and social welfare sectors (cf. Evers & Svetlik, 1993). Public agencies no longer held total responsibility for service provision, but assumed additional accountability for service planning, management, and evaluation. Provision of a continuum of care as well as cost-effectiveness assumed social policy importance equivalent to that in the United States. Case management, or *care management* as it is more frequently termed, appeared to offer solutions to some of the challenges these trends engendered.

It is worth examining snapshot views of case management applications in different countries to see how these forces have played out in different social and cultural contexts. We will see, as well, how familiar issues have surfaced with the implementation of case management, and how other countries are seeking answers to some common dilemmas.

In the United Kingdom in the late 1980s, governmental reports set forth an agenda for case management within systems of community care for the severely mentally ill, the elderly, and disabled adults. Ensuing legislation established block grants consolidating funding for health and social services administered at the local-authority level. Local social service departments were required to purchase services from the "independent" (i.e., voluntary and for-profit) sector, and to focus on assessing care needs. Care managers in local social services departments became the focal point of this system, responsible for need assessments, care planning, service purchasing, budget management, and coordination of care packages. Social service case management teams also provided clinical mental health services, and "key workers" providing case management targeted the most vulnerable clients of mental health authorities (Cox, 1997; Challis & Davies, 1990; Wiener & Cuellar, 1999; Marshall, 1996).

From the start of these programs, problems seen in the U.S. case management experience surfaced (Cox, 1997). Rapidly expanding caseloads and insufficient funding quickly threatened the ability of care managers to meet the objective of having care provided according to need, rather than the services available (Weiner & Cuellar, 1999). Even in areas in which new community care policies have been most developed, services tend to be delivered "off the shelf," and access depends more on social networks and chance than on the activities of case managers (Baldock & Ungerson, 1993, pp. 296, 301). Social service care managers have had to do more with less, picking up areas formerly under the aegis of nurses as other changes in the national health service have cut back both chronic care services and acute care beds. Delegating case management to both social service authorities (for "social aspects" of community care) and health authorities (for the "care programme" for the most vulnerable) threatened to deepen rather than resolve service fragmentation (Holloway, McLean, & Robertson, 1991). This was also the case for the separation of the role of purchaser of services from that of provider, which further placed social workers in potentially adversarial relations with former multidisciplinary teammates (*The Lancet*, 1995). At the budgetary level, allocations have tended to be handled by middle-management care management team leaders. This creates problems both higher and lower in the hierarchy: Lack of knowledge about available funds makes case managers too uncertain about how to plan care, but decentralizing budgetary decisions has also made it hard for social service departments to oversee resource allocation and service development. Nonetheless, at both local and national levels the commitment to community care, and with it case management, has remained secure.

Germany maintained its insistence on a public welfare safety net through the erratic economic and political conditions of the mid to late 1980s (Markovits & Halfmann, 1988). Subsequent to the East-West reunification, a national, non-means-tested social insurance program was enacted. Although different in almost every respect from equivalent systems in England and the United States, this shared an emphasis on community-based care (Weiner & Cuellar, 1999). Austerity budgeting effective in 1997 made considerable cuts in health and pension insurance funds, leading to increased attention to service economies and patient targeting (Grigoleit, 1997). Case management has now become an established feature in services targeted at disabled persons (Gobel, 1999), the elderly (Wissert, 1998), and those with severe mental illness (Walsh & Murray, 1997). The last instance is particularly of interest, since, as in the United States, it was fueled by expectations that outpatient care would replace institutionalization. As in our experience, however, follow-up evaluations have found no significant effects on the rate or duration of hospital stays (Rossler, Loffler, Fatkenheuer, & Riechler-Rossler, 1992, 1995).

Deinstitutionalization was also a major force leading to mental health case management in the Netherlands, with a jump start provided by a review of the U.S. experience by two Dutch researchers (Cox & Broekhuizen, 1989, cited in Willems, 1996). Since the mid-1980s, experiments in case management have also taken place in care for homeless individuals, children of drug addicts, incest survivors, elderly at risk of nursing home placement, the "mentally handicapped," and "intensive home care" for those with serious or terminal illness (Willems, 1996). Issues commonly debated in these efforts include whether case management can fairly be done by direct service providers, the extent of professional expertise required of case managers, and how to deal with threats to provider autonomy. Already driven by policy moves to make care "extramural"(i.e., home- and community-based), case management is now further advanced by attempts to smooth transitions among different sites of care. National policy emphases on cost control and competition are finding place in budgets that are "individual-linked," giving allocation decisions to clients; this too will promote case managers' services, by making them an allowable budget item, and, indirectly, by increasing their use as care consultants.

As these brief views suggest, familiar issues have surfaced with the implementation of case management, regardless of social context. Underlying these common problems are the contradictions introduced by efforts to overcome divisions between purchasing and provider roles, between social services and medical care, and between objectives of effectiveness and efficiency. The forces driving these efforts are now evident around the world. Case management in Australia, widely diffused throughout health and social welfare since its introduction in the mid-1980s, increasingly assumes a brokerage model coordinating purchased services within capitated systems of care (Ozanne, 1996). Although services in Sweden remain primarily public, decentralization and incremental moves toward a mixed system of care have heightened the role of case managers, increasing their caseloads and responsibilities, as well as introducing the "purchaser-provider" model (Hokenstad & Johansson, 1996). Efforts to reform long-term care insurance in Japan center on case managers coordinating community care benefits (Kosaka, 1996), while political commitment to cost-effective resource use in France has prompted specialized case management agencies overseeing negotiations among care providers (Frossard, 1996). In Canadian provinces such as Manitoba, with single-point entry into long-term care systems, case managers have been the fulcrum of care coordination (Berdes, 1996). Now reductions in funding are focusing case management on resource management (Fineman, 1996). Following the devolution of the state welfare system in Croatia, new nonprofit agencies struggle to introduce case management to ensure care of the most vulnerable, as universal benefits are replaced with increased reliance on private and individual responsibility (Jasminka Despot Lucanin, personal communication, Zagreb, June 1999).

Case management worldwide is part of service providers' efforts to stay afloat in the wake of the global economy. The new face of case management draws as well from longstanding tensions in the organization and financing of human services. While it is possible to foresee some degree of isomorphism developing in response to these dynamics, case management structures and practices will also continue to embody their own social and cultural contexts. There is thus much to be learned from studying the similarities and differences emerging in case management around the world. In particular, practice in the United States could be informed by the experiences of countries, such as the United Kingdom, Canada, and Sweden, which have gone further to develop community care, eligibility based on functional rather than financial need, and support for informal caregivers. Case management is in the center of efforts to maintain such priorities while restructuring and retrenching service systems. Identifying the best strategic responses to these pressures could help us use case management to move human services in the United States toward greater equity and effectiveness as well as efficiency.

CONCLUSION

In surveying the institutional and social basis of case management, we have uncovered some remarkable ironies in its structure and operations. Designed as a mechanism to bypass the categorical limitations of service bureaucracies, case management has itself become bureaucratized and hampered by institutional structures. As service sectors have become more specialized and decentralized, the authority of case managers has narrowed, such that many have difficulty accessing services beyond those provided by their particular agency or program area. Insider humor about this condition explores the theme of "how many case managers does it take ..." (Deitchman, 1980) or the vision of clients needing a manager to keep track of their many case managers (Kleyman & Corbett, 1991). One study of mental health services found that case management was the *only* type of program duplicated in the community (Solomon, Gordon, & Davis, 1986).

A second irony is that what is supposed to be a *human link* offering individualized attention from an impersonal system is so typically described and defined in ways that make opaque the personal attributes of all parties involved. As demonstrated previously, this draws from a bureaucratically based claim to status as a service technology; it is fed as well by the scientific attention to the numerical aggregate demanded of program evaluators. It nonetheless seems contradictory for a service with case management's holistic and humanistic objectives to focus only on those aspects of personhood that are related to categories of service need, use, and outcome. What this obscures is the way in which case management is embedded in fundamental elements of the social structure: those which lead women to need and to provide care; those which secure hierarchies of race and class; and those which tie race, class, and gender together.

Given its origins as a tool for enhancing access and advocacy, it may be the ultimate irony for case management itself to reinforce social class inequities. As critics charge, case management may always have been "a myth that has been used to rationalize the current state of fragmentation in the service delivery system" (Moore, 1992, p. 418) or provided "a diversion from under-funding of service programs" (Austin, 1990, p. 402). Now, however, the broader trends shaping case management programs in the United States into two class tiers now may actually increase that fragmentation and reinforce that underfunding, leading to an increased "struggle for fairness between more dominant and less dominant groups" (Stevens & Hall, 1996, cited in Padgett, 1998, pp. 8–9).

Given the interests vested in those trends, it may not be possible to keep case management programs from reflecting the broader social class system. They need not, however, reinforce that system, if they are able to place more emphasis on their underrealized potential for advocacy. From its beginnings, the objectives of case management have included both *case advocacy* to serve and empower particular clients and *class advocacy* to redress problems and deficiencies in service programs and systems (Raiff & Shore, 1993). Both functions are difficult in practice, in part because they can conflict with case managers' development of good working relationships within their local service networks. Thus "the reality is that advocacy is probably the least frequently and least intensively carried out staff activity" (Raiff & Shore, 1993, p. 36).

Through advocacy activities, case management can at least buffer the impact of broader class inequities and introduce countervailing values to challenge the forces generating them. To do so requires more training and support for case managers' skills in "power brokering, effective use of confrontation, risk tolerance . . . resource mobilization and coalition-building" (Raiff & Shore, 1993, p. 57). It further requires administrative finesse and the endowment of case management programs with sufficient clout over fiscal and service resources (Austin, 1990). Through alliances with consumer and other activist groups, as well as the development of peer-modeling programs, case management providers have already prompted many changes affecting people with mental and physical disabilities, people with AIDS, and others (Albrecht & Peters, 1997; Raiff & Shore, 1993). Creative use of its vast symbolic arsenal could help case management remake service systems through change in cultural understandings as well as political action.

NOTES

*The sections of this chapter that precede the international perspectives appeared in a more theoretical treatment in my article, "Case Management as a Cultural Practice," in *Advances in Medical Sociology,* volume 6, pp. 81–117, Gary L. Albrecht, Series Editor, JAI Press, Inc., 1995.

1. See Chapter 1 for discussion of this legislative history.
2. The Omnibus Budget Reconciliation Act (OBRA) of 1981 enabled state Medicaid agencies to obtain a waiver in order to implement programs creating a primary care case manager (typically a physician) who would be the gatekeeper for Medicaid-funded services. Section 2176 of OBRA also authorized waivers for the use of Medicaid funds for community-based (instead of institutional) long-term care; case management was included among the service options for such programs. In 1985, the Consolidated Omnibus Budget Reconciliation Act (COBRA) enabled states to establish primary care case management programs without having to apply for federal waivers. (See Spitz & Abramson, 1987; Applebaum & Austin, 1990.)
3. Case management has even had its own journal, founded as the *Journal of Case Management* by Joan Quinn, one of the early long-term care case management entrepreneurs responsible for initiating the Triage demonstration project (see Chapter 2). The journal still exists, conjoined with *The Journal of Long Term Home Health Care* as *Care Management Journals* (Springer Publishing Company).
4. Among the few pieces of literature analyzing the importance of gender for case management practice are works by Padgett (1998), McAuley, Teaster, and Safewright (1999), and Hasenfeld (1992). See also Mills and Tancred (1992), and especially the article by Grant and Tancred in that volume.

6

Policy for Future Practice

C ase management today is substantially different from its original versions, no matter the sector or program in which it exists. Human services altogether have changed along with profound shifts in political
contexts, social values, and world economies. Before we can see how best
to take case management into the future, we need to understand what and
where it has been in the past and present. This book has examined historically specific applications of case management in order to move toward
that more general understanding.

Several broad themes characterize case management's evolution, each
paralleling trends in social policy. In the sectors we have examined, case
management emerged first in the context of local-level pilot or experimental projects, subsequently achieving success through the sponsorship
of federal initiatives and / or national demonstration programs. These larger-scale applications diffused case management without, however, stan-
dardizing program design or operation. Even those initiatives with strong
programmatic directions that included case management—such as the
Community Mental Health Center Act, the Channeling demonstration, or
the JOBS program—left unspecified many details of implementation. This
was in part political pragmatism, an accommodation to the "political possibilities of the moment" and the contending elements of insider politics,
as Marmor (2000, p. 152) observes of the period's legislative additions to
the Medicare program. It also recognized the necessity of organizational
adaptation to the needs and resources of local service communities. In both
instances, case management offered a bumper cushioning the impact of
federal directives.

Subsequently, control and operation of case management programs returned more completely to the level of states and local governments. This
shift occurred in the context of economic stringency, the rise of procom-
petitive movements in health care and social services, and a loss of faith in
the federal government and the "ameliorative social programs" begun in

the Great Society era (Marmor, 2000, p. 124). Internationally, the spread of case management began as one aspect of the devolution of state authority. These trends made an already variable service mechanism progressively more sensitive and vulnerable to the economics and politics of local contexts. The boundary-spanning nature of case management again made it well suited for this placement. By offering case management, service programs achieved both legitimacy and the ability to gather information on other services and players in their environments. At the same time, acting as "the rear guard in the retreat from big government" (Welch, 1996, p. 1, cited in Austin & McClelland, 1997, p. 120) meant that case managers were doing more with less. What they could do for clients became increasingly and primarily a function of the service resources already available in their local communities. Variability among programs increased, as did the difficulties in demonstrating case management's effectiveness.

Accompanying the move away from the federal level were shifts in the administration of case management from the public realm to quasi-public arrangements, and in turn to the private arena and public/private partnerships. These changes mirrored the fate of the nonprofit sector as it expanded under the "contracting regime" of public sponsorship and dwindled with the ascendance of competitive, market-centered ideologies. By the end of the century, nonprofit service organizations had become largely isomorphic with proprietary ones (Estes, Swan, & Associates, 1993). Corporate interests dominated health care and suffused social welfare. All parties—payers, providers, and clients—were assuming more of the financial risks and burdens of service systems.

The objectives of case management programs show a corresponding change in emphasis over time. When cost containment had been part of early efforts, it was more often as an implicit aspect of other goals (such as deinstitutionalization) than a primary goal itself. The focus (or at least the rhetoric) of those programs was on increasing access to services in the community, with the expectation that care would be cheaper there than in more institutional settings. The failure of such savings to be realized (cf. Weissert, 1985) did not deter those later seeking cost reductions from promoting case management as a valuable tool. Costs of case management programs themselves were curtailed through increased caseloads and de-skilling of workers. Continuing to put a human face on service rationing, case managers filled in gaps in care through their own auspices and ingenuity.

Over the last two decades, social class inequalities have widened to unprecedented levels in this country, while long-standing racial and gender inequalities remain obdurate. Case management programs have sought to redress some of the worst consequences of these inequities. As a long-time analyst notes of wider service integration projects, however, there are inherent limits to an incremental, case-level approach: "However successful individually, [such programs] simply cannot be ginned up to the scale nec-essary to make a dent in the numbers of children and families who need a better shot at success" (Gardner, 1991, p. 16, cited in Kagan & Neville, 1993, p. 176). Yet public policy has abjured radical reform of health care on sev-eral occasions, promoting instead the discipline of the market. Reform of social welfare has inevitably translated into programs promising its demise.

The populations most served by case managers remain those who are both marginal and marginalized within a capitalist economy. Public pro-grams compensate for such limitations and attempt to help people reach a higher rung on the economic ladder, but the ladder too often ends up trun-cated or topped with a glass ceiling. Individuals served within the private realm are those who already have greater privileges of income and ability. Despite other intentions, case management programs continually run the risk of reinforcing the effects of inequitable and unjust systems (Hasenfeld, 2000).

Seeing case management in the context of these broader trends helps us understand the variable forms and contested, contradictory aims it has as-sumed. Constant throughout this time are the vulnerability of the popula-tions case management serves; the categorical nature of service systems it exists in; and the inadequacy of fiscal and service resources to solve the problems at hand. What case management ends up being in practice is a function of many things. Its legislative origins, the professions and other constituencies it involves, its link to fiscal constraint, and social images of its clients are all as responsible for the shape and outcomes of case man-agement as the formal definitions of its structure and goals. One of the few certainties about case management in the future is that it will continue to be a central element of service systems.

For future efforts to be more successful than those of the past requires work on many fronts. Certainly program design and evaluation can bene-fit from such technical enhancements as "crisper units of analysis, clearer statements of the problem, and far clearer specification of outcomes" (Ka-gan & Neville, 1993, p. 175). Developing realistic practice guidelines and identifying the principles of "viable practices that work" are essential steps toward program quality (Kagan & Neville, 1993, p. 188; cf. Geron & Chas-sler, 1994, 1995). Yet it is clear from our historical view that a quest for technical excellence by itself cannot and will not resolve the barriers to the effectiveness of case management programs. If we are to go beyond the technical perfection of an inherently limited practice, we must get to the root of those limitations. Making the most of case management thus re-quires a more critical approach, one that challenges the assumptions that have been its foundation for these several decades. Looking both back-ward and ahead, then, we can identify the following assumptions.

ASSUMPTION 1: CASE MANAGEMENT IS A
NEUTRAL SERVICE TOOL[1]

As it has become more and more integrated within diverse service sectors, case management has achieved an odd form of naturalization. In early forms, program designers treated case management as an experimental black box. The emphasis in program design and evaluation has remained on measuring inputs and outcomes, with considerably less attention to the messier contents of the box itself. Despite or perhaps in counterpoint to case management's intrinsic variability, the emphasis has been, as well, on finding ways to standardize case management programs, in two senses of the term: to reduce the extent to which they vary (beyond what is seen as intentional or useful variation), and to increase the identification and adoption of practice standards. Replication of effective models of case management has been a favored goal of both policy and funding.

As case management programs became an expected part of service delivery to clients with complex care needs, the perspectives embedded in this black box approach became unquestioned elements of the definition of case management. Within such a framework, case management is a neutral tool of service technology, a "strategically benign intervention" enacted in response to self-evident flaws of service systems (Kagan & Neville, 1993, p. 175). The flaw most pointed to by the development of case management programs is a lack of coordination in service delivery. This carries the further implication that service systems are otherwise adequate, appropriate, stable, and available—all assumptions challenged emphatically and repeatedly throughout the last three decades of human service research. Nonetheless, coordination remains a perpetual goal of health care and social service policy, and the more pluralistic the types and control of services, the easier it may be to make political capital of that goal. One reason for case management's success has, in fact, been its tie to a conventionally accepted and politically adaptable problem definition (cf. Marmor, 2000; Austin, 1990).

The problem with treating case management as though it were a neutral tool used in the service of coordination objectives is not so much what this assumption entails, however, as what it excludes. It fails to recognize the values and moral choices embedded in adopting a case management approach as well as in the specifics of program elements. In part, these are part of a program's "practice ideology," its "belief systems about what is 'good' for the client" (Hasenfeld, 1992, p. 13). In turn, these beliefs encompass ideas about who deserves help, what type of help is good, and who should control the definition of terms such as *deserving, help,* and *good.* The issues here pertain as well to broader moral and philosophical questions about the role of case management in social reform. Drawing from a recent assessment of service integration efforts, we must ask, "What do we really expect [case management] to accomplish? Who should define the purposes? Is the emphasis on accessibility, continuity, and efficiency enunciated nearly two decades ago still sufficient today?" (Kagan & Neville, 1993, p. 188).

Viewing case management as a neutral form of service technology also obscures the agency of case managers and of clients. We have seen how case managers actively define the nature of their practice, creatively manipulating or resisting the boundaries of their mandated role. They do this for many reasons: to achieve a practice more in line with their professional training; to make the system work better for clients; or to garner discretion and autonomy (cf. Smith & Lipsky, 1993). Clients, too, "work" the system, and work outside it, to achieve their goals. Together, clients and case managers construct the practice of case management, yet this process of construction is invisible when their actions count only as "noise" or "variability" in a neutral service technology. Such a construction loses information that may be vital to program success, such as the client's understanding of her own life and needs, or the case manager's views of the challenges and satisfactions of her work. Ways in which gender, class, and ethnic relations inform both case management practice and client concerns remain similarly opaque.

The history of case management suggests that it may be neither possible nor desirable to standardize such programs completely. A major strength of these programs, viewed individually or as a subspecies of service organizations, is their adaptability. Case management programs respond to their local contexts, and case managers' practices attune to the philosophies, resources, incentives, and barriers of local service environments. This does not, of course, argue against trying to improve practice standards. It does suggest that such standards, like other program elements, will "transplant" into different contexts only by adapting to them. Understanding that process is vital to our ability to enhance case management's effectiveness.

ASSUMPTION 2: WHAT IS GOOD FOR THE SYSTEM IS GOOD FOR THE CLIENT

We noted in the first chapter that case management objectives exist at both the systems level and that of individual clients, and each case study of a service sector has revealed those dual objectives at work. In the abstract, this is an inevitable concomitant of trying to improve the way systems and programs serve individual clients. In looking at specific case management efforts, however, we have seen how objectives that should be parallel become, in fact, intertwined and confused. Means such as system efficiency become confounded with ends of meeting client needs. *Need* itself is then assessed in terms of what programs can offer clients, and filling available program slots becomes the operational definition of program participation. Programs can be well coordinated yet without substantive meaning in terms relevant to their clients, or they may gain efficiency at the cost of developing meaningful case manager–client relations (cf. Hasenfeld, 2000). The diffusion of case management then occurs through a process within which case management becomes an end in itself, a "standard operating procedure" that defines the range of options operationally available to practitioners and policymakers alike (cf. Marmor, 2000, p. 173).

Separate forms of goal displacement occur when case management strategies favor professional expertise over client perceptions or fail to advocate for clients' individual or collective best interests. In both instances, case managers may unintentionally create or reinforce client dependency. Consumer movements in many service sectors have sought to redress these limitations, but clients differ in the extent and form of control they want to exercise in their service programs. "Empowerment" models need to consider these differences, as well as how definitions and dimensions of what is "empowering" vary for social groups differing in race and ethnicity, age, gender, socioeconomic status, need, and other attributes of social identity (cf. Roberts, 1999).

Absent a context of broader social reform, case management always runs the risk of helping clients adjust and adapt to systems that maintain their vulnerability or oppression. Invoking a "social service orientation" like case management without giving it sufficient flexibility or service resources may only "legitimate the flawed social policy" perpetuating the myth that clients' problems are "personal pathologies" rather than structural in origin (Hasenfeld, 2000, p. 196). Similar risks accrue to defining client needs in the individual terms of human capital approaches, seen particularly in social welfare but more widely as other areas adopt vocational objectives. While augmenting clients' skills, education, and experience should not be undervalued as program goals, there are problems with limiting policy focus to them. One issue is that achieving minimal levels of literacy or education will not overcome a poverty of opportunities for well-paid work (Hasenfeld, 2000). Conversely, education and training may be emphasized only for their contribution to work skills, not their potential for more broadly enhancing the quality of life (Rosenfeld, 2000). Programs thus run the danger of trying to produce "good"and controllable citizens and consumers" (Horsman, 1990, p. 125) rather than helping clients find ways of making life more meaningful as well as productive (cf. Horowitz, 1995).

It is essential that future policy and research clearly differentiate client-centered goals from program- and system-centered ones. To expect case management per se to be an instrument of fundamental social reform would ignore the political, economic, and organizational contexts always shaping its operations. Moreover, case management has now become part of the status quo of service systems. These factors make it even more imperative that we critically assess strategies for achieving change and distinguish outcomes for clients from the means of providing care.

ASSUMPTION 3: CASE MANAGEMENT IS EVERYONE'S RESPONSIBILITY

As case management has multiplied throughout service sectors, it has become incumbent on individual programs to adopt some version of it. Under separate mandates and funding incentives, programs maintain their own case management programs while coordinating with those of others. This, then, becomes a way of perpetuating "service replication ... in the name of service integration" (Kagan & Neville, 1993, p. 167), and making case management everyone's responsibility ensures that it becomes no one's. Clients end up with multiple case managers, but with none of them able to span the entire system of care.

As managed care and other forms of organizational integration contract the networks of providers available to clients, the ability of case managers to coordinate across sector lines becomes increasingly questionable. Also more questionable is the ability of the case manager to act as an advocate for the client rather than as a means of insuring that the services provided are consistent with payer requirements. These reflect in practice the structural ironies Marmor (2000, p. 168) distills from his analysis of managed care's ascendance: "Choice without change, change without choice ..." Current actions countering the power and autonomy managed care organizations have assumed focus on ensuring patients' rights through legislation or litigation. While the legal basis for patient's rights laws is still being contested,[2] if they succeed in being enacted, they will further diffuse accountability to the realm of individual (or class action) advocacy. Whatever benefits might accrue to those individuals, the structure of care will remain unchanged, and the advocacy needs of countless others will remain invisible.

Managed care and service consolidation are also increasingly fixing fiscal accountability for case management programs within the budgets of their parent agencies (cf. Marmor, 2000, pp. 167–168). Yet our knowledge of the problems case management can address, let alone how it can best do so, remains imprecise and partial, at best. Case management programs have always presented formidable challenges to formal evaluations because of their multiple objectives and the many, interacting factors that affect their outcomes (Kagan & Neville, 1993; cf. Weissert, 1985). The costs related to case management programs are notoriously hard to document (Gueron, Pauly, & Lougy, 1991; Davidson, Penrod, Kane, Moscovice, & Rich, 1991; Kane, Penrod, Davidson & Moscovice, 1991), and little work examines the informal costs to individuals and families of care that is not coordinated. These factors again argue for greater attention to the specification and separation of program goals and processes.

At the same time, living up to the responsibility of case management requires more than a technical "fix." Commenting on social welfare, Yeheskel Hasenfeld observes, "The success of any program that aims to change the behavior of its clients depends, first and foremost, on the developing of a trusting relationship between the staff and the clients" (2000, p. 194). This in turn requires "close and frequent contact . . . establishing an empathic relationship; . . . advocating on [clients'] behalf . . . and providing them with personal counseling and support when they are in crisis" (Ibid.). While the specifics will vary in different sectors and with different clients, it is critical that we establish the conditions enabling this type of trusting relationship to develop between case managers and clients. To do otherwise makes assigning responsibility for case management a purely symbolic effort.

CONCLUSION: A REVISION OF CASE MANAGEMENT

Ultimately the best way to use case management is to envision a world where it is no longer necessary. Building on a base and a philosophy of social justice and inclusion, human service programs would organize collaboratively and efficiently. Clients' self-determination and attention to the whole of their lives would be hallmarks of service quality. Trusting relations between human service workers and their clients would be the norm, reinforced by the high value assigned the work of caring for others. Though utopian, these are not, in fact, too far from the highest goals we have always claimed case management programs to have.

The reality of case management has differed from this vision in large part because the claims behind it have been worth so much. It has too often been enough to *have* case management or to use it in the battles of symbolic politics. It has been too easy to use case management programs to reaffirm and reinforce dominant policy paradigms, thus serving purposes of social control rather than social change. The principles inherent in case management have made it effective as a source of white collar employment and service sector expansion: ends some value and others question, but not those of clients. In the name of fiscal accountability, we have too often denied case managers and their programs the conditions most likely to achieve goals for and with the people they serve.

People need more than symbolic services. Still, the hardest symbolic work on case management has yet to be done. We must dare to reconceptualize and reinvent it as a fully human enterprise, not a neutral tool; as a way of fulfilling not just the ends, but the potential of our service programs and professions. We must confront the values that deter us from accepting responsibility for our service systems, in principle and in practice. We have ample opportunity to make case management all that it promises to be, and we owe our future selves no less.

NOTES

1. This discussion owes much to the broader discussion of assumptions in service integration efforts by Kagan and Neville (1993, pp. 161–178) and to comments made by James D. Wright (series editor, letter to Aldine de Gruyter, April 18, 2000).
2. The Supreme Court recently ruled that HMOs cannot be sued in federal court for providing bonuses to physicians to reduce their costs of care, even if withholding care results in harm to a patient. Patients are still able to sue HMOs in federal court for an unjust denial of health benefits. Legislation enabling patients to sue their HMOs in state courts has been enacted recently in several states and introduced in over three dozen state legislatures. ("Supreme Court limits patients' rights," 2000, p. A11). As policy analyst Ted Marmor (2000, p. 167) observes of managed care disputes, "The politics of medicine . . . will be increasingly fought out in state legislatures."

Bibliography

Abel, E. K. (1991). *Who cares for the elderly?* Philadelphia: Temple University Press.

Adams, J. S. (1976). *The structure and dynamics of behavior in organizational boundary roles.* In M. Dunnette (ed.) Handbook of Organizational and Industrial Psychology. Chicago: Rand-McNally.

Adler, M. (1988). *Health and disability status of AFDC families.* 1988 Proceedings of the American Statistical Association: Social Statistics. Alexandria, VA: American Statistical Association.

Administration on Aging. (1995). *1995 state program report for Titles III and VII of the Older Americans Act.* National Aging Program Information System, <http://www.aoa.gov/napis/default.htm>.

Albrecht, G. L., & Peters, K. E. (1995). Organizational theory in the case and care management of health care. *Advances in Medical Sociology, 6,* 1–35.

———. (1997). Peer intervention in case management practice. *Journal of Case Management, 6,* 43–50.

Aldrich, H. E., & Herker, D. (1977). Boundary spanning roles and organizational structure. *Academy of Management Review, 2,* 217–230.

Allen, S., & Mor, V. (1998). *Living in the community with disability: Service needs, use, and systems.* New York: Springer Publishing Co.

Allen, S. M., & Mor, V. (1997). The prevalence and consequences of unmet need. *Medical Care, 35,* 132–148.

Alley, S., Blanton, J., & Feldman, R. E. (Eds.). (1979). *Paraprofessionals in mental health.* New York: Human Sciences Press.

American Public Health Association. (1980). Crisis in the public sector: Challenge to the public's health. *Program and abstracts, 108th Annual Meeting,* Detroit, MI.

Ansak, M. L., & Zawadski, R. (1984). On Lok CCODA: A consolidated model. In R. Zawadski (Ed.), *Community-based systems of long-term care* (pp. 147–170). New York: The Haworth Press.

Applebaum, R. (1996). The case management paradox. *Journal of Case Management, 5,* 90.

Applebaum, R., & Austin, C. (1990). *Long-term care case management: Design and evaluation.* New York: Springer Publishing Company.

Applebaum, R., & Flint, W. (1993). Stuck in adolescence: Will home-care ever come of age? *The Gerontologist, 33,* 278–280.

APWA. (American Public Welfare Association). (1992). *Status report on JOBS case management practices.* Washington, DC: Institute for Family Self-Sufficiency.

———. (1993). *JOBS case management handbook.* Washington, DC: Institute for Family Self-Sufficiency.

———. (1994). *JOBS: Managing JOBS caseloads.* Washington, DC: Institute for Family Self-Sufficiency.

Austin, C. D. (1990). Case management: Myths and realities. *Families in Society, 71,* 398–405.

Austin, C. D., & McClelland, R. W. (1997). Case management in the human services: Reflections of public policy. *Journal of Case Management 6,* 119–126.

Austin, C. D., & O'Connor, K. (1989). Case management: Components and program contexts. In M. D. Peterson & D. L. White (Eds.), *Health Care of the Elderly* (pp. 167–205). Newbury Park, CA:SAGE Publications.

Aviram, U., & Segal, S. P. (1973). Exclusion of the mentally ill: Reflection on an old problem in a new context. *Archives of General Psychiatry, 29,* 126–131.

Aviram, U., Syme, S. L., & Cohen, J. B. (1976). The effects of policies and programs on reduction of mental hospitalization. *Social Science and Medicine, 10,* 571–577.

Axinn, J., & Levin, H. (1997). *Social welfare: A history of the American response to need* (4th edition). New York: Longman Publishers.

Bachrach, L. L. (1976). *Deinstitutionalization: An analytical review and sociological perspective* (U.S. Department of Health, Education, and Welfare Publication No. ADM 76–361). Washington, DC: U.S. Government Printing Office.

Baker, F., & Weiss, R. S. (1984). The nature of case manager support. *Hospital and Community Psychiatry, 35,* 925–928.

Baldock, J., & Ungerson, C. (1993). Consumer perceptions of an emerging mixed economy of care. In A. Evers & I. Svetlik (Eds.), *Balancing pluralism: New welfare mixes in the care of the elderly* (pp. 287–314). Aldershot, UK: Avebury / Ashgate.

Barusch, A. S. (1991). *Caring for the frail elderly: Family support, services, and case management.* New York: Garland.

Batavia, A. I., DeJong, G., & McKnew, L. B. (1991). Toward a national personal assistance program: The Independent Living model of long-term care for persons with disabilities. *Journal of Health Politics, Policy and Law, 16,* 523–545.

Bazeldon Center for Mental Health Law. (1996). *Mental health managed care survey of the states.* Washington, DC: Bazeldon Center for Mental Health Law.

Becker, A., & Schulberg, H. C. (1976). Phasing out state hospitals: A psychiatric dilemma. *New England Journal of Medicine, 294,* 255–261.

Bell, L. V. (1989). From the asylum to the community in U.S. mental health care: A historical overview. In D. A. Rochefort (Ed.), *Handbook on mental health policy in the United States* (pp. 89–120). New York: Greenwood Press.

Bell, W. (1965). *Aid to Dependent Children.* New York: Columbia University Press.

Bell, W. G. (1973). Community care for the elderly: An alternative to institutionalization. *The Gerontologist, 13,* 349–354.

Benjamin, A. E. (1993). An historical perspective on home care policy. *The Milbank Quarterly, 71,* 129–166.

Berdes, C. (1996). Driving the system: Long-term-care coordination in Manitoba, Canada. *Journal of Case Management, 5,* 168–172, 317.

Bernstein, A. G. (1981). Case managers: Who are they and are they making any difference in mental health service delivery? (Doctoral dissertation, University of Georgia, 1981). *Dissertation Abstracts International, 42*, 2125-B-2126-B.

Bertsch, E. (1992). A voucher system that enables persons with severe mental illness to purchase community support services. *Hospital and Community Psychiatry, 43*, 1109–1113.

Binstock, R. H., & Levin, M. A. (1976). The political dilemmas of intervention policies. In R. H. Binstock & E. Shanas (Eds.), *Handbook of aging and the social sciences* (pp. 511–535). New York: Van Nostrand Reinhold.

Blenkner, M., Bloom, M., & Nielson, M. (1971). A research and demonstration project of protective services. *Social Casework, 52*, 483–499.

Bower, K. A. (1992). *Case management by nurses.* Washington, DC: American Nurses Publishing.

Branch, L. G., Coulam, R. F., & Zimmerman, Y. A. (1995). The PACE evaluation: Initial findings. *The Gerontologist, 35*, 349–359.

Brock, T., & Harknett, K. (1998). A comparison of two welfare-to-work case management models. *Social Service Review, 72*, 493–520.

Brodkin, E., & Lipsky, M. (1983). Quality control in AFDC as an administrative strategy. *Social Service Review, 57*, 1–34.

Brown, L. D. (1988). *Health policy in the United States: Issues and options.* Occasional Paper Number Four. Ford Foundation Project on Social Welfare and the American Future. New York: Ford Foundation.

Brown, P. (1985). *The transfer of care: Psychiatric deinstitutionalization and its aftermath.* Boston: Routledge & Kegan Paul.

Burt, M. R., & Pittman, K. J. (1985). *Testing the social safety net.* Washington, DC : The Urban Institute Press.

Burton, J. R. (1994). The evolution of nursing homes into comprehensive geriatrics centers: A perspective. *Journal of the American Geriatrics Society, 42*, 794–796.

Capitman, J. A. (1986). Community-based long-term care models, target groups, and impacts on service use. *The Gerontologist, 26*, 389–397.

Capitman, J. A., Haskins, B., & Bernstein, J. (1986). Case management approaches in coordinated community-oriented long-term care demonstrations. *The Gerontologist, 26*, 398–404.

Carcagno, G. J., & Kemper, P. (1988). The evaluation of the National Long Term Care Demonstration: 1. An overview of the Channeling Demonstration and its evaluation. *Health Services Research, 23*, 1–22.

Carling, P. (1995). *Return to community: Building support systems for people with psychiatric disabilities.* New York: The Guilford Press.

Caton, C. L. M. (1981). The new chronic patient and the system of community care. *Hospital and Community Psychiatry, 32*, 475–478.

Challis, D., & Davies, B. (1986). *Case management in community care.* Aldershot, Hants, England: Gower.

Chamberlain, R., & Rapp, C. A. (1991). A decade of case management: A methodological review of outcome research. *Community Mental Health Journal, 27*, 171–188.

Chandler, S. M. (1990). *Competing realities The contested terrain of mental health advocacy.* New York: Praeger.

Chilman, C. (1992). Welfare reform or revision? The Family Support Act of 1988. *Social Service Review, 66,* 349–377.

Chu, F., & Trotter, S. (1974). *The madness establishment.* New York: Grossman.

Ciosci, H. M., & Goodman, C. L. (1994). A lifetime case management model for persons with spinal cord injury. *Journal of Case Management, 3,* 117–123.

Clark, K. A., Landis, D., & Fisher, G. (1990). The relationship of client characteristics to case management service provision. *Evaluation and Program Planning, 13,* 221–229.

Clemens, E., Wetle, T., Feltes, M., Crabtree, B., & Dubitzky, D. (1994). Contradictions in case management. *Journal of Aging and Health, 6,* 70–88.

Cnaan, R. A. (1994). The new American social work gospel: Case management of the chronically mentally ill. *British Journal of Social Work, 24,* 533–557.

Cohen, E. L., & Cesta, T. G. (1994). Case management in the acute care setting. *Journal of Case Management, 3,* 110–116.

Cohen, R., & Devine, M. (1979). A needs-based service delivery model for community mental health centers. In S. Alley, J. Blanton, & R. Feldman (Eds.), *Paraprofessionals in mental health: Theory and practice* (pp. 203–223). New York: Human Sciences Press.

Conrad, P. (1985). The meaning of medications: Another look at compliance. *Social Science and Medicine, 20,* 29–37.

Cook, F. L., & Barrett, E. J. (1992). *Support for the American welfare state.* New York: Columbia University Press.

Coombs, C., Eisdorfer, C., Feiden, K. L., & Kessler, D. A. (1989). Lessons from the Program for Hospital Initiatives in Long-Term Care. In C. Eisdorfer, D. Kessler, & A. Spector (Eds.), *Caring for the elderly: Reshaping health policy* (pp. 184–196). Baltimore: Johns Hopkins University Press.

Cox, C. (1997). Case management: An American's observations of community care in Britain. *Journal of Case Management, 6,* 88–95.

Curry, J. (1980). A study in case management. *Community Support Service Journal, 2,* 15–17.

Curtis, L. C. (1994). Social integration: Inviting, including, in community. *In Community, 4,* 1–2.

Czerenda, A. J., & Best, L. (1994). Tying it all together. *Journal of Case Management, 3,* 69–73, 87.

Davidson, G. B., Penrod, J. D., Kane, R. A., Moscovice, I. S., & Rich, E. C. (1991). Modeling the costs of case management in long-term care. *Health Care Financing Review, 13,* 73–81.

Davis, I. L. (1992). Client identification and outreach: Case management in school-based services for teenage parents. In B. S. Vourlekis & R. R. Greene (Eds.), *Social work case management* (pp. 27–34). New York: Aldine de Gruyter.

Deegan, P. E. (1992). The Independent Living Movement and people with psychiatric disabilities: Taking back control over our own lives. *Psychosocial Rehabilitation Journal, 15,* 3–19.

Deitchman, W. S. (1980). How many case managers does it take to screw in a lightbulb? *Hospital and Community Psychiatry, 31,* 788–789.

Diamond, T. (1986). Social policy and everyday life in nursing homes: A critical ethnography. *Social Science and Medicine, 23,* 1287–1295.

Dill, A. (1986). *Coordinating care for the elderly: An exploration of organizational process and context* (Doctoral dissertation, Columbia University, 1986). Ann Arbor, MI: University Microfilms International.

———. (1993). Defining needs, defining systems: A critical analysis. *The Gerontologist, 33,* 453–460.

———. (1994). Institutional environments and organizational responses to AIDS. *Journal of Health and Social Behavior, 35,* 349–369.

Dill, A. E. P. (1987). Issues in case management for the seriously mentally ill. In D. Mechanic (Ed.), *Improving mental health services: What the social sciences can tell us. New Directions for Mental Health Services, No. 36* (pp. 61–70). San Francisco: Jossey-Bass.

———. (1990). Transformations of home: The formal and informal process of home care planning. In J. F. Gubrium & A. Sankar (Eds.), *The home care experience* (pp. 227–251). Beverly Hills, CA: Sage Publications.

DiMaggio, P. J., & Powell, W. W.(1991). Introduction. In W. W. Powell & P. J. DiMaggio (Eds.), *The new institutionalism in organizational analysis* (pp. 1–38). Chicago: University of Chicago Press.

Donahue, J. A. (1989). *The privatization decision: Public ends, private means.* New York: Basic Books.

Doolittle, F., & Riccio, J. (1992). Case management in welfare employment programs. In C. F. Manski & I. Garfinkel (Eds.), *Evaluating welfare and training programs* (pp. 310–343). Cambridge, MA: Harvard University Press.

Dorgan, R., & Gerhard, R. (1979). The human service generalist: A framework for integrating and utilizing all levels of staff. In S. Alley, J. Blanton, & R. Feldman (Eds.), *Paraprofessionals in mental health: Theory and practice* (pp. 135–150). New York: Human Sciences Press.

Dorland Healthcare Information. (1999). *Case management resource guide* <http://www.cmrg.com/index.htm> *<cmrg@cmrg.org>* Newport Beach, CA: Author.

Dozier, M., & Franklin, J. (1988). Social disability in the young adult mentally ill. *American Journal of Orthopsychiatry, 58,* 613–617.

Ellison, M. L., Rogers, E. S., Sciarappa, K., Cohen, M., & Forbess, R. (1995). Characteristics of mental health case management: Results of a national survey. *The Journal of Mental Health Administration, 22,* 101–112.

Estes, C. L. (1979). *The aging enterprise.* San Francisco: Jossey-Bass.

———. (1993). The aging enterprise revisited. *The Gerontologist, 33,* 292–298.

Estes, C. L., Swan, J. H., & Associates. (1993). *The long term care crisis.* Newbury Park, CA:SAGE Publications.

Eustis, N. N., & Fischer, L. R. (1992). Common needs, different solutions? Younger and older homecare clients. *Generations, 16,* 17–22.

Evers, A., & Svetlik, I. (Eds.). (1993). *Balancing pluralism: New welfare mixes in the care of the elderly.* Aldershot, England: Avebury/Ashgate.

Federal Register. (1989). *Case management* (§250.43 of the Final Regulations) *54 FR 42146.* Washington, DC.

Fineman, L. (1996). Developing a formal educational program for case managers. *Journal of Case Management, 5,* 158–161.

Fiorentine, R., & Grusky, O. (1990). When case managers manage the seriously mentally ill: A role-contingency approach. *Social Service Review, 64,* 79–93.

Fischer, D. B. (1994). Health care reform based on an empowerment model of re-
    covery by people with psychiatric disabilities. *Hospital and Community Psychi-
    atry, 45*, 913–915.
Fischer, J. (1973). Is casework effective? A Review. *Social Work, 28*, 5–20.
Fisher, G., Landis, D., & Clark, K. (1988). Case management service provision and
    client change. *Community Mental Health Journal, 24*, 134–142.
Foley, H. A. (1975). *Community mental health legislation: The formative process.* Lex-
    ington, MA: Heath.
Frank, R. G., & McGuire, T. G. (1996). Individuals with severe mental illnesses. In
    S. Altman & U. Reinhardt (Eds.), *The Baxter health policy review: Volume II.
    Strategic choices for a changing health care system* (pp. 377–394). Chicago: Health
    Administration Press.
Franklin, J. L. (1988). Case management: A dissenting view. *Hospital and Communi-
    ty Psychiatry, 39*, 921.
Franklin, J. L., Solovitz, B., Mason, M., Clemons, J. R., & Miller, G. E. (1987). An eval-
    uation of case management. *American Journal of Public Health, 77*, 674–678.
Fraser, N., & Gordon, L. (1994). A genealogy of dependency: Tracing a keyword of
    the U.S. welfare state. *Signs: Journal of Women in Culture and Society, 19*, 309–336.
Freidson, E. (1970). *Profession of medicine.* New York: Harper & Row, Publishers.
Freund, D. A., & Neuschler, E. (1986). Overview of Medicaid capitation and case-
    management initiatives. *Health Care Financing Review, 7*, 21–23.
Friday, J. C. (1986). *Case managers for the chronically mentally ill: Assessing and im-
    proving their performance.* Atlanta, GA: Southern Regional Education Board.
Friedland, R., & Alford, R. (1991). Bringing society back in: Symbols, practices, and
    institutional contradictions. In W. W. Powell & P. J. DiMaggio (Eds.), *The new
    institutionalism in organizational analysis* (pp. 232–263). Chicago: The Universi-
    ty of Chicago Press.
Friedman, P. R., & Yohalem, J. B. (1978). The rights of the chronic mental patient. In
    J. A. Talbott, M.D. (Ed.), *The chronic mental patient* (pp. 51–64). Washington, DC:
    The American Psychiatric Association.
Frossard, M. (1996). Case management in France. *Journal of Case Management, 5*,
    162–167.
Gallup, G., Jr. (1994). *The Gallup Poll Public Opinion 1994.* Wilmington, DE: Scholar-
    ly Resources Inc.
Gardner, S. (1991). *Serving children and families effectively: How the past can help chart
    the future.* Washington, DC: Education and Human Services Consortium.
Geertz, C. (1973). *The interpretation of cultures.* New York: Basic Books.
Gelfand, D. E., & Olsen, J. K., with the assistance of Berman, J. (1980). *The aging net-
    work: Programs and services.* New York: Springer Publishing Co.
Gemmill, R. H., Kennedy, D. L., Larison, J. R., Mollerstrom, W. W., & Brubeck,
    K. W. (1992). Case Manager as advocate: Family advocacy in the military. In
    B. S. Vourlekis & R. R. Greene (Eds.), *Social work case management* (pp. 149–165).
    New York: Aldine de Gruyter.
Geron, S. M., & Chassler, D. (1994). The quest for uniform guidelines for long-term
    care case management. *Journal of Case Management, 3*, 91–97.
———. (1995). Advancing the state of the art: Establishing guidelines for long-term
    care case management. *Journal of Case Management, 4*, 9–14.

Gilson, S. F., & Casebolt, G. J. (1997). Personal assistance services and case management. *Journal of Case Management, 6,* 13–17.

Gobel, J. (1999). Case-Management zur erhaltung von arbeitsverhaltnissen behinderter. Ein modellversuch des landesarbeitsamts Bayern. [Case management for maintaining occupational status of handicapped patients. A model trial by the Bavarian federal district office.] *Rehabilitation (Stuttgart), 38,* 209–219.

Goering, P., Durbin, J., Foster, R., Boyles, S., Babiak, T., & Lancee, B. (1992). Social networks of residents in supportive housing. *Community Mental Health Journal, 28,* 199–213.

Goldfinger, S. M., Hopkin, J. T., & Surber, R. W. (1984). Treatment resisters or system resisters?: Toward a better service system for acute care recidivists. In B. Pepper & H. Ryglewicz (Eds.), *Advances in treating the young adult chronic patient. New Directions in Mental Health Services, No. 21* (pp. 17–27). San Francisco: Jossey-Bass.

Gordon, L. (1994). *Pitied but not entitled.* New York: The Free Press.

Gorey, K. M., Leslie, D. R., Morris, T., Carruthers, W. V., John, L., & Chacko, J. (1998). Effectiveness of case management with severely and persistently mentally ill people. *Community Mental Health Journal, 34,* 241–250.

Granet, R. B., & Talbott, J. A. (1978). The continuity agent: Creating a new role to bridge the gaps in the mental health system. *Hospital and Community Psychiatry, 29,* 132–133.

Grau, L. (1984). Case management and the nurse. *Geriatric Nursing, 5,* 372–375.

Greenberg, J. N., Leutz, W. N., & Altman, S. H. (1989). The Social Health Maintenance Organization. In C. Eisdorfer, D. Kessler, & A. Spector (Eds.), *Caring for the elderly: Reshaping health policy* (pp. 197–223). Baltimore: The Johns Hopkins University Press.

Greenblatt, M., & Richmond, S. S. (1979). *Public welfare, notes from underground.* Cambridge, MA: Schenkman.

Greene, R. R. (1992). Case management: An arena for social work practice. In B. S. Vourlekis & R. R. Greene (Eds.), *Social work case management* (pp. 11–25). New York: Aldine de Gruyter.

Grigoleit, H. (1997). Einsparpotentiale in der rehabilitation—durch gezieltere patientenauswahl. [Economizing potential in rehabilitation—through targeted patient selection.] *Rehabilitation (Stuttgart), 36,* 7–11.

Grob, G. N. (1991). *From asylum to community:Mental health policy in modern America.* Princeton, N J: Princeton University Press.

———. (1994). Government and mental health policy: A structural analysis. *The Milbank Quarterly, 72,* 471–499.

Gronfein, W. (1985). Incentives and intentions in mental health policy: A comparison of the Medicaid and Community Mental Health Programs. *Journal of Health and Social Behavior, 26,* 192–206.

Grusky, O., Tierney, K., Holstein, J., Anspach, R., Davis, D., Unruh, D., Webster, S., Vandewater, S., & Allen, H. (1985). Models of local mental health delivery systems.—*in W. R. Scott & B. L. Black (eds.), The organization of mental health services* (pp.159–195). Beverly Hills, CA: SAGE Publications.

Gueron, J. M., & Pauly, E., with Lougy, C. M. (1991). *From welfare to work.* New York: Russell Sage Foundation.

Haber, C., & Gratton, B. (1994). *Old age and the search for security.* Bloomington, IN: Indiana University Press.

Hagen, J. (1994). JOBS and case management: Developments in 10 states. *Social Work, 39,* 197–205.

Hagen, J. L. (1999). Public welfare and human services: New directions under TANF? *Families in Society: The Journal of Contemporary Human Services, 80,* 78–90.

Hagen, J. L., & Davis, L. V. (1994). *Implementing JOBS: The participants' perspective.* Albany, NY: The Nelson A. Rockefeller Institute of Government.

Hagen, J. L., & Lurie, I. (1994a). *Implementing JOBS: Case management services.* Albany, NY: The Nelson A. Rockefeller Institute of Government.

———. (1994b). *Implementing JOBS: Progress and promise.* Albany, NY: The Nelson A. Rockefeller Institute of Government.

Haines, D. W. (1990). Conformity in the face of ambiguity: A bureaucratic dilemma. *Semiotica, 78,* 249–269.

Hamilton, W. L., Burstein, N. R., Hargreaves, M., Moss, D. A., & Walker, M. (1993). *The New York State Child Assistance Program: Program impacts, costs and benefits.* Cambridge, MA: Abt Associates, Inc.

Hamner, K., & Bryant, D. (1997). Do client characteristics predict case management activity? *Evaluation and Program Planning, 20,* 259–267.

Handelman, D., & Leyton, E. (1978). *Bureaucracy and world view.* Memorial University of Newfoundland, Institute of Social and Economic Research, Social and Economic Studies No. 22. Toronto: University of Toronto Press.

Handler, J. F., & Hasenfeld, Y. (1991). *The moral construction of poverty: Welfare reform in America.* Newbury Park, CA: Sage Publications.

Hansell, N., Wodarczyk, M., & Visotsky, H. M. (1968). The mental health expediter. *Archives of General Psychiatry, 18,* 392–396.

Hargreaves, M. B. (1993). *The New York State Child Assistance Program: Program implementation.* Cambridge, MA: Abt Associates, Inc.

Harris, M., Bergman, H. C., & Greenwood, V. (1982). Integrating hospital and community systems for treating revolving-door patients. *Hospital and Community Psychiatry, 33,* 225–227.

Hasenfeld, Y. (1972). People processing organizations: An exchange approach. *American Sociological Review, 37,* 256–263.

———. (1992). The nature of human service organizations. In Y. Hasenfeld (Ed.), *Human services as complex organizations* (pp. 3–23). Newbury Park, CA: SAGE Publications.

———. (2000). Social services and Welfare-to-Work: Prospects for the social work profession. *Administration in Social Work, 23,* 185–199.

Hasenfeld, Y., & Weaver, D. (1996). Enforcement, compliance, and disputes in Welfare-to-Work programs. *Social Service Review, 70,* 235–256.

Hegar, R. L. (1992). Monitoring child welfare services. In B. S. Vourlekis & R. R. Greene (Eds.), *Social work case management* (pp. 135–148). New York: Aldine de Gruyter.

Henderson, M. G., Souder, B A., Bergman, A., & Collard, A. F. (1988). Private sector initiatives in case management. *Health Care Financing Review,* 1988 Annual Supplement, 89–95.

Herr, T., & Halpern, R. (1994). *Lessons from Project Match for welfare reform.* Chicago: Project Match, Erikson Institute.

Herzfeld, M. (1992). *The social production of indifference.* Chicago: The University of Chicago Press.

Hoge, M. A., Davidson, L., Griffith, E. E. H., Sledge, W. H., & Howenstine, R. A. (1994). Defining managed care in public-sector psychiatry. *Hospital and Community Psychiatry, 45,* 1085–1089.

Hokenstad, M. C., & Johansson, L. (1996). Eldercare in Sweden: Issues in service provision and case management. *Journal of Case Management, 5,* 137–141.

Hokenstad, M. C., Jr. (1982). Introduction. In M. C. Hokenstad, Jr., & R. A. Ritvo (Eds.), *Social service delivery systems: An international annual: Vol. 5. Linking health care and social services. International perspectives* (pp. 11–24). Beverly Hills, CA: Sage Publications.

Holloway, F., McLean, E. K., & Robertson, J. A. (1991). Case management. *British Journal of Psychiatry, 159,* 142–148.

Honnard, R. (1985). The chronically mentally ill in the community. In M. Weil, J. M. Karls, & Associates (Eds.), *Case management in human service practice* (pp. 204–232). San Francisco: Jossey-Bass.

Hopper, K., Baxter, E., & Cox, S. (1982). Not making it crazy: The young homeless patients in New York City. In B. Pepper & H. Ryglewicz (Eds.), *The young adult chronic patient. New Directions for Mental Health Services, No. 14* (pp. 33–42). San Francisco: Jossey-Bass.

Horowitz, R. (1995). *Teen mothers: Citizens or dependents?* Chicago: The University of Chicago Press.

Horsman, J. (1990). *Something in my mind besides the everyday: Women and literacy.* Toronto: Women's Press.

Hromco, J. G., Lyons, J. S., & Nikkel, R. E. (1995). Mental health case management: Characteristics, job function, and occupational stress. *Community Mental Health Journal, 31,* 111–125.

———. (1997). Styles of case management: The philosophy and practice of case managers. *Community Mental Health Journal, 33,* 415–428.

Hurley, R. E., & Fennell, M. L. (1990). Managed-care systems as governance structures: A transaction-cost interpretation. In S. S. Mick & Associates (Eds.), *Innovations in health delivery: Insights for organization theory* (pp. 241–268). San Francisco: Jossey-Bass.

Huxley, P., & Warner, R. 1992. Case management, quality of life, and satisfaction with services of long-term psychiatric patients. *Hospital and Community Psychiatry, 432,* 799–802.

In Profile. (1994). Debra Anderson. *In Community, 4,* 5.

Intagliata, J., & Baker, F. (1983). Factors affecting case management services for the chronically mentally ill. *Administration in Mental Health, 11,* 75–91.

James, V. (1979). Paraprofessionals in mental health: A framework for the facts. In S. Alley, J. Blanton, & R. E. Feldman (Eds.), *Paraprofessionals in mental health: Theory and practice* (pp. 19–37). New York: Human Sciences Press.

JCAH (Joint Commission on Accreditation of Hospitals). (1976). *Principles for accreditation of Community Mental Health Service programs.* Chicago: JCAH.

Johnson, P. J., & Rubin, A. (1983). Case management in mental health: A social work domain? *Social Work, 28,* 49–55.

Kagan, S. L., with Neville, P. R. (1993). *Integrating families for children and families: Understanding the past to shape the future.* New Haven, CT: Yale University Press.

Kahana, E., & Coe, R. M. (1975). Alternatives in long-term care. In S. Sherwood (Ed.), *Long term care: A handbook for researchers, planners, and providers* (pp. 511–572). New York: Spectrum Publications.

Kane, R. A. (1988). The noblest experiment of them all: Learning from the National Channeling Evaluation. *Health Services Research, 23,* 189–198.

Kane, R. A., & Caplan, A. L. (Eds.). (1993). *Ethical conflicts in the management of home care: The case manager's dilemma.* New York: Springer.

Kane, R. A., & Kane, R. L. (1987). *Long-term care: Principles, programs, and policies.* New York: Springer.

Kane. R. A., Penrod, J. D., Davidson, G., & Moscovice, I. (1991). What cost case management in long-term care. *Social Service Review, 65,* 281–303.

Kane, R. A., Penrod, J. D., & Kivnick, H. Q. (1994). Case managers discuss ethics: Dilemmas of an emerging occupation in long-term care in the United States. *Journal of Case Management, 3,* 3–12.

Kaplan, K. O. (1990). Recent trends in case management. *Encyclopedia of Social Work* (18th edition), 60–77. Silver Spring, MD: National Association of Social Workers.

Karger, H. J. (1983). Reclassification: Is there a future in public welfare for the trained social worker? *Social Work, 38,* 427–433.

Katz, M. (1986). *In the shadow of the poor house.* New York: Basic Books.

Kemper, P. (1988). The evaluation of the National Long Term Care Demonstration: 10. Overview of the findings. *Health Services Research, 23,* 161–174.

Kemper, P., Applebaum, R., & Harrigan, M. (1987). Community care demonstrations: What have we learned? *Health Care Financing Review, 8,* 87–100.

Kleinman, A. (1978). Concepts and a model for the comparison of medical systems as cultural systems. *Social Science and Medicine, 12,* 85–93.

Klerman, G. (1977). Better but not well: Social and ethical issues in the deinstitutionalization of the mentally ill. *Schizophrenia Bulletin, 3,* 617–631.

Kleyman, P., & Corbett, J. (1991). Cartoon showing older person in bed, surrounded by case managers and saying over the phone, "Marge, I think I'll need a manager to keep track of all my care managers!" *Aging Today,* December 1991 / January 1992, p. 9.

Korr, W. S., & Cloninger, L. (1991). Assessing models of case management: An empirical approach. *Journal of Social Service Research, 14,* 129–161.

Kosaka, M. (1996). Developing a health service system for the elderly in Japan. *Journal of Case Management, 5,* 182–185.

Kosterlitz, J. (1989). Devil in the details. *National Journal,* Dec. 2, 2942–2946.

LaFond, J. Q., & Durham, M. L. (1992). *Back to the asylum: The future of mental health law and policy in the United States.* New York: Oxford University Press.

Lamb, H. R. (1980). Therapist-case managers: More than brokers of services. *Hospital and Community Psychiatry, 31,* 762–764.

———. (1981). What did we really expect from deinstitutionalization? *Hospital and Community Psychiatry, 32,* 105–109.

———. (1986). Some reflections on treating schizophrenics. *Archives of General Psychiatry, 43,* 1007–1011.

Lamb, H. R., & Talbott, J. A. (1986). The homeless mentally ill. The perspective of the American Psychiatric Association. *JAMA, 256,* 498–501.

The Lancet. (1995). Editorial. Care-management: A disastrous mistake. *345*, 399–401.

Larson, M. S. (1977). *The rise of professionalism: A sociological analysis.* Berkeley, CA: University of California Press.

Lefley, H. P. (1996). Impact of consumer and family advocacy movements on mental health services. In B. L. Levin & J. Petrila (Eds.), *Mental health services: A public health perspective* (pp. 81–96). New York: Oxford University Press.

Lens, V., & Pollack, D. (1999). Welfare reform: Back to the future! *Administration in Social Work, 23*, 61–77.

Leutz, W., Sciegaj, M., & Capitman, J. (1997). Client-centered case management: A survey of state programs. *Journal of Case Management, 6*, 18–24.

Levine, I. S., & Fleming, M. (1986). *Human resource development: Issues in case management.* Manpower Development Unit and Community Support Project, State of Maryland Mental Hygiene Administration.

Levine, M., Tulkin, S., Intagliata, J., Perry, J., & Whitson, E. (1979). The paraprofessional: A brief social history. In S. Alley, J. Blanton, & R. E. Feldman (Eds.), *Paraprofessionals in mental health: Theory and practice* (pp. 38–71). New York: Human Sciences Press.

Lipsky, M. (1984). Bureaucratic disentitlement in social welfare programs. *Social Service Review, 58*, 3–27.

Lloyd, P. (1991). The empowerment of elderly people. *Journal of Aging Studies, 5*, 125–135.

Love, R. (1984). The Community Support Program: Strategy for reform? In J. A. Talbott (Ed.), *The chronic mental patient: Five years later* (pp. 195–214). Orlando, FL: Grune and Stratton.

Lowery, S. L. (1995). *Case management in Skilled Nursing Facilities: An administrative and clinical guide to successful implementation.* Presentation to the Massachusetts Extended Care Federation on April 18, 1995.

Lubove, R. (1975). *The professional altruist: The emergence of social work as a career 1880–1930.* New York: Atheneum.

Lupton, D. (1994). *Medicine as culture: Illness, disease and the body in Western societies.* Thousand Oaks, CA: Sage Publications.

MacAdam, M., Capitman, J., Yee, D., Prottas, J., Leutz, W., & Westwater, D. (1989). Case management for frail elders: The Robert Wood Johnson Foundation's Program for Hospital Initiatives in Long-Term Care. *The Gerontologist, 29*, 737–744.

Mahoney, K. J., & Simon-Rusinowitz, L. (1997). Cash and Counseling Demonstration and Evaluation: Start up activities. *Journal of Case Management, 6*, 25–30.

Markovits, A. S., & Halfmann, J. (1988). The unraveling of West German social democracy? In M. K. Brown (Ed.), *Remaking the Welfare State* (pp. 96–188). Philadelphia: Temple University Press.

Marmor, T. R. (2000). *The politics of Medicare.* New York: Aldine de Gruyter.

Marmor, T. R., & Rein, M. (1973). Reforming "the welfare mess": The fate of the Family Assistance Plan, 1969–72. In A. P. Sindler (Ed.), *Policy and politics in America* (Chapter 1). Boston: Little, Brown.

Marshall, M. (1996). Case management: A dubious practice. *BMJ, 312*, 523–524.

Maynard, R. (Ed.). (1993). *Building self-sufficiency among welfare-dependent teenage parents.* Princeton, NJ: Mathematica Policy Research, Inc.

McAuley, W. J., Teaster, P. B., & Safewright, M. P. (1999). Incorporating feminist ethics into case management programs. *Journal of Applied Gerontology, 18,* 3–24.

McGreevy, M. A. (1986). A profile of New York State's CSS case managers. *Community Support Services* (The New York State Office of Mental Health, The Evaluation Research Unit), *1,* 1–4.

Mechanic, D. (1980). *Mental health and social policy* (2nd edition). Englewood Cliffs, NJ: Prentice Hall.

———. (1986). The challenge of chronic mental illness: A retrospective and prospective view. *Hospital and Community Psychiatry, 37,* 891–896.

Meyer, J. W., & Rowan, B. (1977). Institutionalized organizations: Formal structure as myth and ceremony. *American Journal of Sociology, 83,* 340–363.

Meyer, J. W., Scott, W. R., & Deal, T. E. (1981). Institutional and technical sources of organizational structure: Explaining the structure of educational organizations. In H. D. Stein (Ed.), *Organization and the human services: Cross disciplinary reflections* (pp. 151–179). Philadelphia: Temple University Press.

Miller, N. (1992). Plan implementation and coordination: Case management in an Employee Assistance Program. In B. S. Vourlekis & R. R. Greene (Eds.), *Social work case management* (pp. 125–134). New York: Aldine de Gruyter.

Miller, N. A. (1992). Medicaid 2176 Home and Community-Based Care Waivers: The first ten years. *Health Affairs, 11,* 162–171.

Mills, A. J., & Tancred, P. (Eds.). (1992). *Gendering organizational analysis.* Newbury Park, CA: Sage Publications.

Mishler, E. G., Amarasingham, L. R., Osherson, S. D., Hauser, S. T., Waxler, N. E., & Liem, R. (Eds.). (1981). *Social contexts of health, illness, and patient care.* New York: Cambridge University Press.

Moore, S. (1992). Case management and the integration of services: How service delivery systems shape case management. *Social Work, 37,* 418–423.

Mor, V., Fleishman, J. A., Allen, S. M., & Piette, J. D. (1994). *Networking AIDS services.* Ann Arbor, MI: Health Administration Press.

Morris, R. (1981). Foreword. In D. L. Frankfather, M. J. Smith, & F. G. Caro (Eds.), *Family care of the elderly* (pp. ix–xvi). Lexington, MA: Lexington Books.

Mueser, K. T., Bond, G. R., Drake, R. E., & Resnick, S. G. (1998). Models of community care for severe mental illness: A review of research on case management. *Schizophrenia Bulletin, 24,* 37–73.

Mullahy, C. A. (1996). Case management and managed care. In P. R. Kongstvedt (Ed.), *The Managed health care handbook* (3rd edition) (pp. 274–300). Washington, DC: Aspen Publishers, Inc.

Mundinger, M. O. (1983). *Home care controversy: Too little, too late, too costly.* Rockville, MD: Aspen Systems Corporation.

NAPGCM (National Association of Professional Geriatric Care Managers). (1992). *Standards of practice for professional geriatric care managers.* Phoenix, AZ: NAPGCM.

NASW (National Association of Social Workers). (1992). *NASW standards for social work case management.* Washington, DC: NASW.

———. (1997). *Social work speaks*. Washington, DC: NASW.

Nathanson, C. A. (1977). Sex, illness, and medical care: A review of data, theory, and method. *Social Science and Medicine, 11*, 13–25.

National Conference on Social Welfare. Task Forces on the Organization and Delivery of Human Services: The public, private, and consumer partnership. (1976). *Expanding management technology and professional accountability in social service programs: Final report*. Columbus, OH: Author.

National Conference on Social Welfare. Task Forces on the Organization and Delivery of Human Services. (1977). *The future for social services in the United States. Final report of the task force*. Columbus, OH: Author.

National Conference on Social Welfare. (1981). *Final report. Case management: State of the art*. Submitted to U.S. Department of Health and Human Services, April 15. Columbus, OH: Author.

National Institute of Mental Health. (1982). *A network for caring: The Community Support Program of the National Institute of Mental Health*. Washington, DC: U.S. Department of Health and Human Services, Public Health Service, Alcohol, Drug Abuse, and Mental Health Administration.

Netting, F. E., Warrick, L. H., Christianson, J. B., & Williams, F. G. (1994). Determinants of client termination in hospital-based case management programs. *Journal of Case Management, 3*, 74–80.

Nightingale, D. S., Wissoker, D. A., Burbridge, L. C., Bawden, D. L., & Jeffries, N. (1991). *Evaluation of the Massachusetts Employment and Training Choices Program: Final results and implications for JOBS*. Washington, DC: Urban Institute Press.

1971 White House Conference on Aging. (1971). *Toward a national policy on aging: Final report*. Washington, DC: U.S. Government Printing Office.

Noble, C. (1997). *Welfare as we knew it*. New York: Oxford University Press.

O'Connor, G. G. (1988). Case management systems and practice. *Social Casework, 69*, 97–106.

Older Americans Act of 1978. (1978). Hearings before the Subcommitee on Aging of the Committee on Human Resources, United States Senate, Ninety-fifth Congress, Second Session on S. 2850. Washington, DC: U.S. Docs.

O'Neill, J. (1990). *Work and welfare in Massachusetts: An evaluation of the ET Program*. Boston: Pioneer Institute for Public Policy Research.

Osgood, K. (1992). *Loneliness among persons with serious mental illness: A re-analysis of existing data*. Unpublished master's thesis, University of Wisconsin–Stout.

Ozanne, E. (1996). Case management applications in Australia. *Journal of Case Management, 5*, 153–157.

Padgett, S. M. (1998). Dilemmas of caring in a corporate context: A critique of nursing case management. *Advancing in Nursing Sciences, 20*, 1–12.

Pecora, P. J., & Austin, M. J. (1983). Declassification of social service jobs: Issues and strategies. *Social Work, 28*, 421–426.

Pepper, B., Kirshner, M. C., & Ryglewicz, H. (1981). The young adult chronic patient: Overview of a population. *Hospital & Community Psychiatry, 32*, 463–469.

Pepper, B., & Ryglewicz, H. (Eds.). (1982). *The young adult chronic patient. New directions for mental health services, No. 14*. San Francisco: Jossey-Bass.

Perlman, N. (1976). Hospital employees' perspective on deinstitutionalization. In
    V. Bradley (Ed.), *Paper victories and hard realities* (pp. 39–44). Washington, DC:
    Georgetown University Health Policy Center.
Perlmutter, F. D. (1997). *From welfare to work.* New York: Oxford University Press.
Pescosolido, B. A., Wright, E. R., & Sullivan, W. P. (1995). Communities of care: A
    theoretical perspective on case management models in mental health. *Advances in Medical Sociology, 6,* 37–79.
Pfeiffer, E. (1973). Introduction to the Conference Report. In E. Pfeiffer (Ed.), *Alternatives to institutional care for older Americans: Practice and planning—A Conference Report.* Durham, NC: Duke University Center for the Study of Aging and
    Human Development.
Phillips, B. R., Kemper, P., & Applebaum, R. A. (1988). The evaluation of the National Long Term Care Demonstration: 4. Case management under Channeling. *Health Services Research, 23,* 67–81.
Piette, J., Fleishman, J. A., Mor, V., & Dill, A. (1990). A comparison of hospital and
    community case management programs for persons with AIDS. *Medical Care, 28,* 746–755.
Piliavin, I., & Gross, A. E. (1977). The effects of separation of services and income
    maintenance on AFDC recipients. *Social Service Review, 51,* 389–406.
Piven, F. F., & Cloward, R. A. (1993). *Regulating the Poor: The Functions of Public Welfare* (updated edition). New York: Vintage Books.
Platman, S. R., Dorgan, R. E., Gerhard, R. S., Mallam, K. E., & Spiliadis, S. S. (1982).
    Case management of the mentally disabled. *Journal of Public Health Policy, 3,* 302–314.
Popple, P., & Reid. P. N. (1999). A profession for the poor? A history of social work
    in the United States. In G. R. Lowe & P. N. Reid (Eds.), *The Professionalization of Poverty* (pp. 9–28). New York: Aldine de Gruyter.
Pratt, H. J. (1976). *The gray lobby.* Chicago: University of Chicago Press.
The President's Commission on Mental Health. (1978). *President's Commission on Mental Health Report.* Washington, DC: U.S. Government Printing Office.
Quadagno, J. S. (1988). *The transformation of old age security: Class and politics in the American welfare state.* Chicago: University of Chicago Press.
Quinn, J. (1994). Case management in a changing world. *Journal of Case Management, 3,* 90, 109.
Quinn, J. L., & Hodgson, J. H. (1984). Triage: A long term care study. In R. T. Zawadski (Ed.), *Community-based systems of long term care* (pp. 171–194). New
    York: The Haworth Press.
Rabin, D. L., & Stockton, P. (1987). *Long-term care for the elderly: A factbook.* New York:
    Oxford University Press.
Raiff, N. R., with Shore, B. K. (1993). *Advanced case management: New strategies for the 90s.* Newbury Park, CA: Sage Publications.
Rapp, C. A. (1998). The active ingredients of effective case management: A research
    synthesis. *Community Mental Health Journal, 34,* 363–380.
Rapp, C. A., & Chamberlain, R. (1985). Case management services for the chronically mentally ill. *Social Work, 30,* 417–422.
Rapp, C. A., & Kisthardt, W. (1996). Case management with people with severe and
    persistent mental illness. In C. D. Austin & R. W. McClelland (Eds.), *Perspec-*

tives in case management practice (pp. 17–45). Milwaukee, WI: Families International, Inc.

Read, W. A., & O'Brien, J. L. (1989). The involved hospital. In C. Eisdorfer, D. A. Kessler, & A. N. Spector (Eds.), *Caring for the elderly: Reshaping health policy* (pp. 157–183). Baltimore: Johns Hopkins University Press.

Reich, R. (1973). Care of the chronically mentally ill: A national disgrace. *American Journal of Psychiatry, 130,* 911–912.

Reif, R., & Reissman, F. (1965). The indigenous nonprofessional. *Community Mental Health Journal, Monograph Series, Number 1.*

Reverby, S. M. (1987). *Ordered to care: The dilemma of American nursing—1850–1945.* Cambridge, MA: Cambridge University Press.

Riccio, J., Friedlander, D., & Freedman, S., with Farrell, M. E., Fellerath, V., Fox, S., & Lehman, D. (1994). *GAIN: Benefits, costs and three-year impacts of a welfare-to-work program.* New York: Manpower Demonstration Research Corporation.

Riccio, J., Goldman, B., Hamilton, G., Martinson, K., & Orenstein, A. (1989). *GAIN: Early implementation experiences and lessons: California's Greater Avenues for Independence Program.* New York: Manpower Demonstration Research Corporation.

Ridgely, M. S., Morrissey, J. P., Paulson, R. I., Goldman, H. H., & Calloway, M. O. (1996). Characteristics and activities of case managers in the RWJ Foundation Program on Chronic Mental Illness. *Psychiatric Services, 47,* 737–743.

Roberts, K. J. (1999). Patient empowerment in the United States: A critical commentary. *Health Expectations, 2,* 82–92.

Rochefort, D. A. (1986). *American social welfare policy.* Boulder, CO: Westview Press.
———. (1989). Mental illness and mental health as public policy concerns. In D. A. Rochefort (Ed.), *Handbook on mental health policy in the United States* (pp. 3–20). New York: Greenwood Press.
———. (1993). *From poorhouses to homelessness: Policy analysis and mental health care.* Westport, CT: Auburn House.
———. (1997). *From poorhouses to homelessness: Policy analysis and mental health care* (2nd edition). Westport, CT: Auburn House.

Rochefort, D. A., & Dill, A. E. P. (1994). Moving welfare recipients toward self-sufficiency through improved case management. In L. Brown & K. Ciffolillo (Eds.), *Invitation to change: Better Government Competition on Welfare Reform 1994 Winners* (pp. 61–79). Boston: Pioneer Institute for Public Policy Research.

Rodeheaver, D. (1987). When old age became a social problem, women were left behind. *The Gerontologist, 27,* 741–746.

Rose, S. (1979). Deciphering deinstitutionalization: Complexities in policy and program analysis. *Milbank Memorial Fund Quarterly, 37,* 429–461.

Rosen, A. L., Pancake, J. A., & Rickards, L. (1995). Mental health policy and older Americans: Historical and current perspectives. In M. Gatz (Ed.), *Emerging issues in mental health and aging* (pp. 1–18). Washington, DC: American Psychological Association.

Rosenfeld, L. (2000). *The implications of an integrative lens in human service organization and program design: Factors of ethnicity, social class, gender, and literacy.* Unpublished Senior Honors Thesis, Brown University.

Rossler, W., Loffler, W., Fatkenheuer, B., & Riechler-Rossler, A. (1992). Does case management reduce the rehospitalization rate? *Acta Psychiatrica Scandinavica, 86,* 445–449.

———. (1995). Case management for schizophrenic patients at risk for rehospitalization: A case control study. *European Archives of Psychiatry and Clinical Neuroscience, 246,* 29–36.

Rowe, M. (1992). Is case management effective for people with serious mental illness? A research review. *Health and Social Work, 17,* 138–150.

———. (1999). *Crossing the border.* Berkeley: University of California Press.

Sabatino, C. P., & Litvak, S. (1992). Consumer-directed home care: What makes it possible? *Generations, 16,* 53–57.

Satinsky, M. A. (1995). *An executive guide to case management strategies.* Chicago: American Hospital Publishing, Inc.

Scala, M. A., Mayberry, P. S., & Kunkel, S. R. (1996). Consumer-directed home care: Client profiles and challenges. *Journal of Case Management, 5,* 91–99.

Schmidt-Posner, J., & Jerrell, J. M. (1998). Qualitative analysis of three case management programs. *Community Mental Health Journal, 34,* 381–392.

Schneider, B. W., Hirsch, C., Galper, M. K., Rickards, S. W., & Sterthous, L. M. (1984). *A year in the lives of clients and case managers.* Department of Health, Education, and Welfare (DHEW) Contract 90-AR-0004A/01. Philadelphia: Temple University Institute on Aging.

Schram, B., & Mandell, B. R. (1997). *An introduction to human services policy and practice.* Boston: Allyn and Bacon.

Schwartz, S. R., Goldman, H. H., & Churgin, S. (1982). Case management for the chronic mentally ill: Models and dimensions. *Hospital and Community Psychiatry, 33,* 1006–1009.

Scott, W. R. (1981). Reform movements and organizations: The case of aging. In S. B. Kiesler, J. N. Morgan, & V. K. Oppenheimer (Eds.), *Aging: Social change* (pp. 331–344). New York: Academic Press.

———. (1991). Unpacking institutional arguments. In W. W. Powell & P. J. DiMaggio (Eds.), *The new institutionalism in organizational analysis* (pp. 164–182). Chicago: University of Chicago Press.

Scott, W. R., & Backman, E. V. (1990). Institutional theory and the medical care sector. In S. S. Mick & Associates (Eds.), *Innovations in health care delivery* (pp. 20–52). San Francisco: Jossey-Bass.

Scott, W. R., & Meyer, J. W. (1991). The organization of societal sectors: Propositions and early evidence. In W. W. Powell & P. J. DiMaggio (Eds.), *The new institutionalism in organizational analysis* (pp. 108–140). Chicago: University of Chicago Press.

Scull, A. T. (1976). The decarceration of the mentally ill: A critical view. *Politics and Society, 6,* 173–211.

Secord, L. J. (1987). *Private case management for older persons and their families.* Elcelsior, MN: Interstudy.

SEIU (Service Employees International Union) Local 509, Welfare Chapter (n.d.). Welfare department with welfare reform. Case management staff. Financial assistance social worker series.

Selznick, P. (1957). *Leadership in administration.* Evanston, IL: Row, Peterson.

Sheets, J. L., Prevost, J. A., & Reihman, J. (1982). Young adult chronic patients: Three hypothesized sub-groups. *Hospital and Community Psychiatry, 33,* 197–203.

Sherwood, S. (1975). Long-term care: Issues, perspectives and directions. In S. Sherwood (Ed.), *Long term care: A handbook for researchers, planners, and providers* (pp. 3–79). New York: Spectrum.

Siegal, H. A. (Ed.). (1994). The application of case management in the treatment of drug and alcohol abuse. *Journal of Case Management, 3* (Special Issue).

Simon-Rusinowitz, L., & Hofland, B. F. (1993). Adopting a disability approach to home care services for older adults. *The Gerontologist, 33,* 159–162.

Smith, S. R., & Lipsky, M. (1993). *Nonprofits for hire: The welfare state in the age of contracting.* Cambridge, MA: Harvard University Press.

Smith, S. R., & Stone, D. A. (1988). The unexpected consequences of privatization. In M. K. Brown (Ed.), *Remaking the welfare state* (pp. 232–252). Philadelphia: Temple University Press.

Sobey, F. (1970). *The nonprofessional revolution in mental health.* New York: Columbia University Press.

Solomon, P. (1992). The efficacy of case management services for severely mentally disabled clients. *Community Mental Health Journal, 28,* 163–179.

Solomon, P., B. Gordon, B., & Davis, J. M. (1986). Reconceptualizing assumptions about community mental health. *Hospital and Community Psychiatry, 37,* 708–712.

Spitz, B. (1987). A national survey of Medicaid Case-Management Programs. *Health Affairs, 6,* 61–70.

Spitz, B., & Abramson, J. (1987). Competition, capitation, and case management: Barriers to strategic reform. *The Milbank Quarterly, 65,* 348–370.

Starr, P. (1982). *The social transformation of American medicine.* New York: Basic Books.

Stassen, M., & Holahan, J. (1981). *Long-term care demonstration projects: A review of recent evaluations.* Washington, DC: The Urban Institute.

Stein, L. I., & Test, M. A. (1978). An alternative to mental hospital treatment. In L. I. Stein & M. A. Test (Eds.), *Alternatives to mental hospital treatment* (pp. 43–55). New York: Plenum.

Steiner, G. Y. (1966). *Social insecurity: The politics of welfare.* Chicago: Rand McNally and Company.

———. (1971). *The state of welfare.* Washington, DC: The Brookings Institution.

Stroul, B. A. (1984). *Toward Community Support Systems for the mentally disabled: The NIMH Community Support Program.* Boston: Center for Rehabilitation Research and Training in Mental Health.

———. (1986). *Models of Community Support Services: Approaches to helping persons with long-term mental illness.* Boston: Center for Psychiatric Rehabilitation.

Subcommittee on Aging, Committee on Human Resources, United States Senate, Ninety-Fifth Congress, Second Session. (1978). Hearings on S. 2850 to amend the Older Americans Act to provide for improved programs for the elderly and for other purposes and related bills. U.S. Docs.

Sullivan, J. P. (1981). Case Management. In J. A. Talbott (Ed.), *The chronic mentally ill: Treatment, programs, systems* (pp. 118–131). New York: Human Sciences Press.

"Supreme Court limits patients' rights to sue HMOs over bonuses," *The Providence Journal,* June 13, 2000, p. A11.

Swidler, A. (1986). Culture in action: Symbols and strategies. *American Sociological Review, 51,* 273–286.

Task Panel of the President's Commission on Mental Health. (1978). Report on de-institutionalization, rehabilitation, and long-term care. In *Task Panel's Reports submitted to The President's Commission on Mental Health, Vol. II Appendix* (pp. 356–375). Washington, DC: U.S. Government Printing Office.

The Technical Committee on Physical and Mental Health with the collaboration of A. B. Chinn, E. S. Colby, & E. G. Robins. (1971). *1971 White House Conference on Aging, Physical and Mental Health.* Washington, DC: White House Conference on Aging.

TenHoor, W. J. (1982). United States: Health and personal social services. In M. C. Hokenstad, Jr., & R. A. Ritvo (Eds.) *Social service delivery systems: An international annual: Vol. 5. Linking health care and social services International perspectives* (pp. 25–59). Beverly Hills, CA: Sage Publications.

Tessler, R. C., Goldman, H. H., & Associates. (1982). *The chronically mentally ill: Assessing Community Support Programs.* Cambridge, MA: Ballinger Publishing Company.

Test, M. A., & Stein, L. I. (1976). Practical guidelines for the community treatment of markedly impaired patients. *Community Mental Health Journal, 12,* 72–82.

Testimony of Stephen B. Heintz, Commissioner of the Connecticut Department of Income Maintenance and Chairman of APWA Matter of Commitment Steering Committee on behalf of the American Public Welfare Association and its project "Investing in poor families and their children: A matter of commitment," before the Finance Subcommittee on Social Security and family policy Washington, DC, January 23, 1987. Washington, DC: American Public Welfare Association.

Thompson, K. S., Griffith, E. E., & Leaf, P. J. (1990). A historical review of the Madison model of community care. *Hospital and Community Psychiatry, 41,* 625–634.

Torres-Gil, F. (1992). *The new aging: Politics and change in America.* Westport, CT: Auburn House.

Trainor, J., Shepherd, M., Boydell, K. M., Leff, A., & Crawford, E. (1997). Beyond the service paradigm: The impact and implications of consumer/survivor initiatives. *Psychiatric Rehabilitation Journal, 21,* 132–140.

Treas, J. (1995). Older Americans in the 1990s and beyond. *Population Bulletin, 50,*No. 2.

Treffert, D. A. (1983). The dollar follows the patient, not the dollars. In J. A. Talbott (Ed.), *Unified mental health systems: Utopia unrealized. New Directions for Mental Health Services, No. 18* (pp. 33–37). San Francisco: Jossey-Bass.

Turner, J. C., & TenHoor, W. J. (1978). The NIMH Community Support Program: Pilot approach to a needed social reform. *Schizophrenia Bulletin, 4,* 319–349.

U.S. General Accounting Office. (1977). *Returning the mentally disabled to the community: Government needs to do more.* HRD-76–152. Washington, DC: Author.

———. (1993). *Long-term-care case management: State experiences and implications for federal policy.* GAO/HRD-93–52. Washington, DC: Author.

———. (1994a). *Medicaid long-term care: Successful state efforts to expand home services while limiting costs.* GAO/HEHS-94–167. Washington, DC: Author.

———. (1994b). *Long-term care reform: States' views on key elements of well-designed programs for the elderly.* GAO/HEHS-94–227. Washington, DC: Author.

————. (1997). *Welfare reform: States' early experiences with benefit termination.* Washington, DC: Author.

U.S. Senate, Committee on Finance. (1987). Welfare: Reform or Replacement? (Child Support Enforcement). Statement of Dorothy V. Harris, ACSW, President, National Association of Social Workers. S. Hrg. 100–335.

Vogel, R. J., & Palmer, H. C. (1985). *Long-term care: Perspectives from research and demonstrations.* Rockville, MD: Aspen Systems Corporation.

Vourlekis, B. S. (1992). The policy and professional context of case management practice. In B. S. Vourlekis & R. R. Greene (Eds.) *Social work case management* (pp. 1–9). New York: Aldine de Gruyter.

Wallack, S. S. (1991). Managed care: Practice, pitfalls, and potential. *Health Care Financing Review, 12,* 27–34.

Walsh, E., & Murray, R. M. (1997). Does case management influence the rate of violence and self-destructive behaviours in the severely mentally ill? *International journal of psychiatry in clinical practice, 1,* 95–100.

Weaver, D., & Hasenfeld, Y. (1997). Case management practices, participants' responses, and compliance in Welfare-to Work programs. *Social Work Research, 21,* 92–100.

Weber, M. (1978). *Economy and society* (2nd edition). G. Roth & C. Wittick (Eds. and Trans.). Berkeley, CA: University of California Press.

Weil, M. (1985a). Key components in providing services. In M. Weil, J. M. Karls, & Associates (Eds.), *Case management in human service practice* (pp. 29–71). San Francisco: Jossey-Bass.

————. (1985b). Professional and educational issues in case management practice. In M. Weil, J. M. Karls, & Associates (Eds.), *Case management in human service practice* (pp. 357–390). San Francisco: Jossey-Bass.

Weil, M., & Karls, J. M. (1985). Historical origins and recent developments. In M. Weil, J. M. Karls, & Associates (Eds.), *Case management in human service practice* (pp. 1–28). San Francisco: Jossey-Bass.

Weissert, W. G. (1985). Seven reasons why it is so difficult to make community-based long-term care cost effective. *Health Services Research, 20,* 423–433.

Weissert, W. G. (1988). The National Channeling Demonstration: What we knew, know now, and still need to know. *Health Services Research, 23,* 175–187.

Weissert, W. G., Cready, C. M., & Pawelak, J. E. (1988). The past and future of home- and community based long-term care. *The Milbank Quarterly, 66,* 309–388.

Welch, B. (1996). Case management in context: Policies and politics. *Plenary session presentation at the Third International Conference on Long Term Care Case Management.* San Diego, CA.

Westermeyer, J. (1988). Response from Dr. Westermeyer. *American Journal of Public Health 78,* 93–94.

White, M., & Grisham, M. (1982). *The structure and processes of case management in California's Multipurpose Senior Services Project.* Berkeley, CA: University of California at Berkeley.

White, M., Gundrum, G., Shearer, S., & Simmons, W. J. (1994). A role for case managers in the physician office. *Journal of Case Management, 2,* 62–68.

White House Conference on Aging. (1961). *Aging in the states: A report of progress, concern, goals.* Washington, DC: U.S. Government Printing Office.

———. (1981). *Final report. The 1981 White House Conference on Aging: Vol. 2. Process proceedings.* Washington, DC: U.S. Government Printing Office.

Wiener, J. M., & Cuellar, A. E. (1999). Public and private responsibilities: Home- and community-based services in the United Kingdom and Germany. *Journal of Aging and Health, 11,* 417–444.

Wilensky, H. L., & Lebeaux, C. N. (1965). *Industrial society and social welfare.* New York: Free Press.

Willems, D. (1996). The case manager in Holland: Behind the dikes. *Journal of Case Management, 5,* 146–152.

Wimberley, E. T., & Blazyk, S. (1989). Monitoring patient outcome following discharge: A computerized geriatric case-management system. *Health and Social Work, 14,* 269–276.

Wissert, M. (1998). Grundfunktionen und fachliche standards des unterstutzungs-managements. [Basic functions and specialty standards of support management.] *Zeitschrift Fur Gerontologie und Geriatrie, 31,* 332–337.

Wyers, N. L. (1980.) Whatever happened to the income maintenance line worker? *Social Work, 35,* 259–263.

Yordi, C. L. (1988). Case management in the social health maintenance organization demonstrations. *Health Care Financing Review,*1988 Annual Supplement, 83–88.

Zawadski, R. T. (1984a). The Long Term Care Demonstration Projects: What are they and why they came into being. In R. T. Zawadski (Ed.), *Community based systems of long term care* (pp. 5–19). New York: The Haworth Press.

———. (1984b). Research in the demonstrations: Findings and issues. In R. T. Zawadski (Ed.), *Community based systems of long term care* (pp. 209–228). New York: The Haworth Press.

Zawadski, R. T., & Eng, C. (1988). Case management in capitated long-term care. *Health Care Financing Review, 9,* 75–81.

Zlotnik, J. L. (1996). Case management in child welfare. In C. D. Austin & R. W. McClelland (Eds.), *Perspectives in case management practice* (pp. 47–72). Milwaukee, WI: Families International, Inc.

Zucker, L. G. (1991). The role of institutionalization in cultural persistence, postscript: Microfoundations of institutional thought. In W. W. Powell & P. J. DiMaggio (Eds.), *The new institutionalism in organizational analysis* (pp. 103–107). Chicago: University of Chicago Press.

Index

Bureaucracy (*cont.*)
   tion of client to, 157–158; representation to client, 158; rise of, 8

Canada, case management in, 170
Capitalism, effect on case manage-
   ment, 167, 171
Care management, 168
Care management journals, 173 n.3
Care mapping, 47
Care plan development, 5
Caregiver respite services, 33
Caregivers: effect of services and bene-
   fits on, 73 n.11; response to services and benefits, 43
Case advocacy, 172
Case finding, for elderly, 32
Case identification, 5
Case-level approach, limits of, 176–177
Case management: adaptability of, 45;
   as black box, 25–26, 36, 53; capital-
   istic objectives of, 167; client goals,
   6–7; client outcomes of, 43; comparison of models, 41–44; constituencies of, 153 (*see also* Clients);
   consumer responsibility for, 52;
   cost outcomes of, 43; as cultural
   tool, 160–162; current forms of,
   17–18, 165–166; definitions of, 4–
   5; deprofessionalization of, 132
   (*see also* Paraprofessionals); effectiveness of, 2–3; efficacy of, 150–
   152, 155–156; evaluations of, 39,
   150–151; evolution of, 11–14, 175;
   expansion of, 3; familistic sides of,
   164; federal mandate of, 15–16;
   foundation support of, 15; in institutional settings, 47–48; legitimization of, 41, 56; local and state
   autonomy in, 15–16, 55 (*see also*
   Local governments; State governments); nature of, 42, 156; objectives of, 5, 14; OBRA incentives
   for, 40; origins of, 7–8; as part of
   broader policies, 152–153; policy
   objectives, 44–45, 54–55, 156; professionalization of, 53, 56; pro-

grammatic goals of, 45–46; responsibility for, 181–182; revenue
   sources, 13; service coordination
   component (*see* Service coordination) service system goals, 6–7; as
   service technology, 54–56, 178–
   179; standardization, resistance to,
   2, 155–156, 179; symbolic importance, 157; technology of, 5; utility
   of, 153–154; variability in, 54–55
Case Management Institute, 51
Case management practice, 57–69; administrative tasks, 98; case definition, 60, 63; case management
   roles, 99; client assessments, 98;
   client-caregiver–service provider
   relationship management, 60–61;
   client dependency status, 66–67,
   101; client-homemaker relationship management, 59–60, 62, 65;
   client relationship building, 103;
   clinical perspective, 65–66; conflicts of interest in, 67–68; consumer-directed programs, 103–
   104; contradictions within, 94–95;
   cultural competency and sensitivity issues, 164–165; elements of
   practice, variability in, 98; guidelines for, 177; methodology implementation, overlap in, 97;
   multidisciplinary approach of, 64;
   needs assessment, 65; and policy
   objectives, disconnect with, 161;
   referrals for services, 61; relations
   with other agencies, 59, 61, 63; services, unbundling, 61–62; system-
   driven nature of, 98–99
"Case Management Resource Guide,"
   167
Case managers, 5, 17; administrative
   pressures on, 162; authority of,
   171; as boundary-spanners, 22; in
   BSS programs, 84; and clients, relationship with, 182; differences in
   practice, 161–162; ethical dilemmas, 70; as human link, 5, 158,
   171–172; for mental health care,